ROUTLEDGE LIBRARY EDITIONS:
WOMEN IN SOCIETY

Volume 4

MAN-MADE WOMEN

MAN-MADE WOMEN

How New Reproductive Technologies Affect Women

GENA COREA, RENATE DUELLI KLEIN, JALNA HANMER, HELEN B. HOLMES, BETTY HOSKINS, MADHU KISHWAR, JANICE RAYMOND, ROBYN ROWLAND AND ROBERTA STEINBACHER

Routledge
Taylor & Francis Group
LONDON AND NEW YORK

First published in 1985 by Hutchinson and Co. (Publishers) Ltd

This edition first published in 2025
by Routledge
4 Park Square, Milton Park, Abingdon, Oxon OX14 4RN

and by Routledge
605 Third Avenue, New York, NY 10158

Routledge is an imprint of the Taylor & Francis Group, an informa business

British Library Cataloguing in Publication Data
A catalogue record for this book is available from the British Library

ISBN: 978-1-032-87216-2 (Set)
ISBN: 978-1-032-85086-3 (Volume 4) (hbk)
ISBN: 978-1-032-85094-8 (Volume 4) (pbk)
ISBN: 978-1-003-51650-7 (Volume 4) (ebk)

DOI: 10.4324/9781003516507

Publisher's Note
The publisher has gone to great lengths to ensure the quality of this reprint but points out that some imperfections in the original copies may be apparent.

Disclaimer
The publisher has made every effort to trace copyright holders and would welcome correspondence from those they have been unable to trace.

Man-Made Women

How new reproductive technologies affect women

Gena Corea, Renate Duelli Klein, Jalna Hanmer,
Helen B. Holmes, Betty Hoskins, Madhu Kishwar,
Janice Raymond, Robyn Rowland and
Roberta Steinbacher

Hutchinson

London Melbourne Sydney Auckland Johannesburg

Hutchinson and Co. (Publishers) Ltd

An imprint of the Hutchinson Publishing Group

17–21 Conway Street, London W1P 6JD

Hutchinson Publishing Group (Australia) Pty Ltd
16–22 Church Street, Hawthorn, Melbourne, Victoria 3122

Hutchinson Group (NZ) Ltd
32–34 View Road, PO Box 40–086, Glenfield, Auckland 10

Hutchinson Group (SA) (Pty) Ltd
PO Box 337, Bergvlei 2012, South Africa

First Published 1985

Set in 11 on 12 point Plantin by J&L Composition Ltd,
Filey, North Yorkshire

Printed and bound in Great Britain by
Anchor Brendon Ltd,
Tiptree, Essex

British Library Cataloguing in Publication Data

Man-made women: how new reproductive technologies
affect women.—(Explorations in feminism; 10)
1. Human reproduction—Social aspects
2. Medical innovations—Social aspects
I. Corea, Gena II. Series
306′.46 QP251

ISBN 0 09 162731 1

Contents

Notes on contributors

Gena Corea is a journalist and has lectured extensively on women's health and reprotechnology. She is the author of *The Hidden Malpractice: How American Medicine Mistreats Women* (1977, reprinted 1985) and *The Mother Machine: Reproductive Technologies from Artificial Insemination to Artificial Wombs* (1985).

Renate Duelli Klein is a neurobiologist and researcher in women's studies. Together with Rita Arditti and Shelley Minden she has edited *Test-Tube Women. What Future for Motherhood?* (1984). She is one of the editors of *Women's Studies International Forum* and the *Athene Series*: An International Collection of Feminist Books.

Jalna Hanmer is a sociologist and co-ordinates the MA in women's studies at Bradford University. She researches and writes on violence to women and reproductive technology and together with Sheila Saunders has published *Well-Founded Fear: A community study of violence to women* (1984).

Helen Bequaert 'Becky' Holmes is a biologist with special interests in population genetics, human biology, and bioethics. With Betty B. Hoskins and Michael Gross she edited *Birth Control and Controlling Birth: Women-Centred Perspectives* (1980) and *The Custom-Made Child* (1981). She is currently studying reproductive technologies in the Netherlands.

Betty Hoskins was educated as a developmental and molecular biologist and now works as a senior technical editor at a computer company. She has been interested in the issue of reproductive technology for a long time and edited two books on the subject together with Becky Holmes and Michael Gross (see under Holmes).

Madhu Kishwar teaches literature at Delhi University and is working on her Ph.D. thesis on the nineteenth-century women's reform movements in India. She is a founder member and editor of *Manushi: A Journal About Women and Society*.

Janice Raymond is associate professor of women's studies and medical ethics at the University of Massachusetts in Amherst, USA. She is the author of *The Transsexual Empire: The Making of the She-Male* (1979) and *Female Friendship: A Philosophy* (forthcoming 1986).

Robyn Rowland is a social psychologist and lecturer in women's studies at Deakin University, Australia. She has researched the social and psychological consequences of human artificial insemination. She has also edited *Women Who Do and Women Who Don't Join the Women's Movement* (1984) and two books of poetry: *Filigree in Blood* (1982) and *Rainbow Warrior* (forthcoming).

Roberta Steinbacher is a social psychologist and professor of Urban Studies at Cleveland State University in Ohio, USA. Presently she is on leave as an Administrator of the Ohio Bureau of Employment Services.

Preface

Janice Raymond

The essays collected in this volume originated as presentations at the 2nd International Interdisciplinary Congress on Women in Groningen, Holland in April 1984. The panel, entitled 'The Death of the Female', was organized to represent feminist perspectives on the new reproductive technolgies (RTs), emphasizing sex predetermination, but including *in vitro* fertilization (IVF), surrogate motherhood, and embryo transfer. Co-organized and chaired by Becky Holmes (USA) and Robyn Rowland (Australia) the panel represented an international group of women thinkers, writers, and activists who had worked in the reproductive technology area for some time: Gena Corea (USA), Renate Duelli Klein (Switzerland, now living in London), Roberta Steinbacher (USA), Madhu Kishwar (India), and Janice Raymond (USA).

The title of this panel reflects the urgent and life-threatening dimensions that these technologies pose for women. So too do the essays in this book. But they also represent much more than yet another form of women's oppression. They highlight the emerging feminist concerns about the new RTs as well as some of the actions that women on an international scale have taken on these issues.

An important action that emerged from the panel presentation in Groningen was the founding of a new 'Feminist International Network on the New Reproductive Technologies' (FINNRET). Since April of 1984, the network membership has grown to over 500 members. Its aims are: to monitor developments in the areas of reproductive engineering; to assess the implications of the new reproductive technologies, such as surrogate motherhood and artificial insemination, on the position and well-being of women internationally; to bring together members of the network periodically to pool information, strategize, and develop policies for women's groups to consider and discuss; and to educate women globally about the interaction of technology, population policy, and feminist goals. FINNRET also seeks to involve women in the decision-making processes concerned with health, population, and social welfare processes within their own countries. Ultimately, its goals are to *educate* and to *empower* women. Like the network, the essays in this book seek not only to enlighten but to empower.

Becky Holmes and Betty Hoskins lay out very clearly the technologies now being used and researched in the area of sex predetermination. Madhu Kishwar provides an example of the practical application of these technologies in portraying the situation of women, and the proliferation of clinics for sex selection, in India. The brothel model that Gena Corea uses in her analysis illustrates on another graphic level the actual conditions that do exist and that could be further implemented to control the 'fabrication' of life. What is important to understand here is that not only is fetal life being fabricated – to which traditional ethicists and policy makers will object – but *female* life is being molded as well. The emphasis on test-tube babies is misleading to the extent that it obscures the medical creation of 'test-tube women'; women whose bodies and minds are used as 'living laboratories', as 'mother machines', and who are thus subjected to yet another form of exploitation.*

Roberta Steinbacher and Becky Holmes summarize the data on gender preference – the fact that son preference exists universally in almost every culture. I would add to their important research that sex preference for boy children is not an isolated phenomenon. It exists on a continuum in which preference for men, from heterosexuality to sex predetermination of one's children, has been a value world-wide. We must view son preference, and the technologies being developed to implement the preference, in a wider context.

To Renate Duelli Klein's title-question, 'What's "new" about the

---

* This phrase was taken from the title of *Test-Tube Women: What Future for Motherhood?*, edited by Rita Arditti, Renate Duelli Klein, and Shelley Minden (London and Boston: Pandora Press 1984). 'Living laboratories' is Robyn Rowland's term and 'mother machine' the title of Gena Corea's recent book (1985).

"new" reproductive technologies?', I would answer a new form of female victimization – *previctimization*, i.e. the oppression and obliteration of the female before she is born. Duelli Klein's essay also emphasizes the important connections between the old and new reproductive technologies in such a way that we see how 'old' the 'new' technologies really are while at the same time what is distinctly 'new' about their import for women.

Robyn Rowland focuses on the issue of *choice* in the sex predetermination context. She asks the important question: 'What of a "choice" which closes opportunities to women as a social group?' *Voluntarism* has been used over and over again as a camouflage for more subtle forms of coercion. In the reproductive technologies domain, we see it operating in statements such as 'infertile women want *in vitro* technology', or 'parents have the right to choose the sex of their child'. What is rarely discussed is how the whole social context not only conditions a woman's choices but her *motivation* to choose as well. This is what one might want to call a voluntaristic means of behaviour control and modification.

Lastly, Jalna Hanmer explores the question to what extent we are now faced with yet another appropriation of women's lives. In the same way medical experts and sexologists have been busy defining women's sexuality over the last hundred years,* today it is women's *reproduction* that is being technologically manipulated to a yet unprecedented degree and thus gradually removed from our control. Hanmer's piece was added to the conference papers, and by making it the last contribution in this collection, we hope the reader will close this book with the desire to reflect on the multifaceted nature of the threat these technologies pose for women, and with the determination to act on this knowledge.

The potential for the control of reproduction under the guise of its being benevolent, voluntaristic, and therapeutic, is enormous. It has already begun in the technologies that these essays discuss. However, control here has entered with a whimper, not with a bang. And conformity, the conformity of women once again to new forms of old reproductive roles (what scientists are now calling 'protected

* For an analysis see Lal Coveney *et al.*, *The Sexuality Papers* (London: Hutchinson 1984).

pregnancies') is being enforced in the name of therapy and choice, at the individual's request, and with the effect of satisfied consumers of the 'therapy'.

Perhaps the most confusing message about the new reproductive technologies is that they are a gift to women, because they appear to give so-called infertile women the ability to reproduce. However, when women look this 'gift-horse' in the mouth, they will see that it comes accompanied by the persistent *medicalization* of women's lives. This means that more and more areas of female living have been colonized by medical intervention, and staked out as medical territory. The medicalization of female existence, begun with the nineteenth-century establishment of the specialities of gynaecology and obstetrics, becomes outrageously solidified in the new technologies of reproduction. Obscured by all the recent accounts of the 'miracles' of reproductive technologies is the immense amount of biomedical probing, manipulation, and experimentation to which women who seek out such 'wonders' of technological fertility and birthing are subject.

Surrounded by such 'gifts', women must ask from whence they come. Why do these fabulous medical techniques require that women adapt to the most painful and debilitating circumstances? Why do such technologies reinforce the bio-medical 'fact' that a woman's reproductive system is pathological and requires an enormous amount of bio-intervention? Why do these techniques reduce the totality of a woman's being to that which is medically manipulatable? Under the cover of a new science of reproduction, how is the female body being fashioned into the biological laboratory of the future? And finally, will the ultimate feat of these technologies be to remove not only the control of reproduction, but reproduction itself, from women? These essays make clear that the engineering of human reproduction, and the forms it has taken, could only occur in a society where the anti-feminist dimensions of the technologies run deeper than is apparent at first glance.

Indeed, these essays do make it clear that the anti-feminist dimensions are entrenched in the ideologies, treatment, and bio-medical promises that spawn the proliferation of the new reproductive technologies. This does not mean that the anti-feminism of the 'technodocs'* and their reproductive engineering proposals are always intentional, planned, or conspiratorial. It was Hannah Arendt who gave us the concept of the 'banality of evil'.† It is not bio-medical monsters or conspiracies that necessarily engineer the abuse, maiming, or previctimization of increasing numbers of women. Antifeminism can be extreme without possessing demonic, or designed dimension. Many 'technodocs' do not wrong women because they are ontologically evil, monstrous, or conspiring. Things are not all that simple. Each of these essays reveals the *complexity* of the new reproductive technologies discussion.

Montague, USA
December 1984

---

* The word is Gena Corea's. See *The Mother Machine* (New York: Harper & Row 1985).

† See Hannah Ahrendt, *Eichmann in Jerusalem. A report on the banality of evil* (New York : The Viking Press, revised edition 1965).

1 Prenatal and preconception sex choice technologies: a path to femicide?

Helen B. Holmes and Betty B. Hoskins

Introduction

One of nature's well-kept secrets has long been the sex of the unborn human child. But people have always pried into nature's secrets ... and this secret is no exception. We shall discuss what scientists have learned about nature's ways of sex determination; how veterinary and medical technologists have attempted to influence that determination; how clinical technologists have attempted to identify sex before birth; why researchers do this work; and what the grave implications are for all women. Indeed, attempts to choose the sex of our children may reveal deep sexist, racist, and classist biases.

In humans, sex is determined at the moment of conception, when the sperm merges with the egg, usually as the egg is passing down one of the fallopian tubes. Each human egg contains twenty-three chromosomes; one of these is the X-chromosome. Each human sperm also contains twenty-three chromosomes: one of these is either an X *or* a Y. The sperm fertilizes the egg, bringing the chromosome count to forty-six and starting either a female (XX) or a male (XY) offspring. A photograph of a cell's chromosomes, preserved at the division stage and stained with a dye, can be used to prepare a 'karyotype' for chromosome identification.

Because the Y-chromosome is much smaller than the X; there is 3.5 per cent less DNA (the main component of chromosomes) in a Y-bearing sperm. And, when stained with the dye quinacrine, a Y-chromosome usually contains a spot (the F-body) that fluoresces under ultraviolet light or a laser beam.

Sperm separation

An obvious way to control sex is to concentrate or to remove either X-sperm or Y-sperm from a sample of semen. Various methods are used in biochemistry laboratories to separate tiny particles with somewhat dissimilar properties from each other; many of these have been tried with semen samples (Ericsson and Glass 1982)*. As yet no method works adequately, as judged by independent observers, despite inventors' own claims.

Cattle breeders have a strong financial incentive to get a good sperm separation technique; most cattle today are conceived by artificial insemination. For dairy, only females are needed; for beef, only males are wanted. One American ranch owner, Ericsson, has patented a sperm separation method which produces a sample enriched in non-defective Y-sperm, leaving the X-sperm and defective sperm behind (Ericsson 1977), and which, he says, works better with human than with bull sperm. He has authorized the use of his patent for human sex selection in clinics at seven locations in the USA, which advertised 'for sex selection (male) and male infertility'. In Ericsson's report in 1982, 75 per cent of ninety-one children were male (Beernink and Ericsson 1982).

Although at present no technique exists that everyone agrees really works, much research effort is going on; some effective method of sperm separation will very likely soon be worked out. Though most of this work is in the beef-eating USA, some is in Belgium (by Indonesians) and in Germany (where Ericsson first tried his method). (See references in Adimoelja *et al.* 1977; Ericsson and Glass 1982; Steeno *et al.* 1975.)

Other methods of influencing which kind of sperm will fertilize the egg are under investigation around the world. Excess of one sex here or there in history, or in specific locations, has been correlated with factors such as diet, minerals in drinking water, sexual practices that restrict intercourse to specific times in a woman's menstrual cycle, low or high sperm count within the female tract, and the timing of artificial insemination (Guttentag and Secord 1982, pp. 100–10). Twentieth-century gynaecologists have sometimes suggested certain

---

* Full references quoted in the text are contained in the references sections at the end of chapters.

behavioural practices to their patients; one or another may be derived from a folk practice that perhaps has a biological basis. Some have been reported in such widely circulated medical journals as the *New England Journal of Medicine* (e.g. Guerrero 1974; Harlap 1979). We started our research into the literature on these behavioural methods as total sceptics; however, there might be a bit of fire under all the smoke, since women's knowledge is largely undocumented.

The effect of diet, one revival of an old folk idea, has recently been described in several medical journals by Dr Stolkowski from Paris and Dr Lorrain from Montreal. To conceive a boy, Stolkowski and Lorrain say, the potential mother should eat, for the preceeding six weeks, foods high in sodium and potassium; for a girl, foods high in calcium and magnesium (Lorrain and Gagnon 1975; Langendoen and Proctor 1982; Stolkowski and Choukroun 1981; Stolkowski and Duc 1977). Theoretical explanations propose that the woman's internal mineral balance may affect the cervical mucus through which sperm must travel, or the fallopian tube up which sperm must swim, or the 'zona pellucida' around her egg's membrance (Debrovner 1982). Proof, however, is lacking.

Also proposed as a factor that may influence which type of sperm fertilizes the egg is the sperm count within the female tract. A healthy man has a high sperm count after he abstains from intercourse for a few days; low sperm counts may result from poor nutrition, radiation, drugs, environmental chemicals, or frequent intercourse. 'Research suggests tentatively that increased frequency [of intercourse] for the female (especially near ovulation) produces more male conceptions, while high frequency for the male, with his wife only occasionally a partner, leads to more female conceptions' (Guttentag and Secord 1983: p. 105). The implication is that girls are conceived when men are undernourished or fickle! And again, solid experimental evidence does not exist.

Sex detection

What have scientists done to uncover the well-kept secret of the sex of the already conceived, but as yet unborn, offspring? Of the many different methods under investigation, one, indeed, is essentially 100 per cent reliable. Many people know about this technique: amniocentesis, followed by karyotyping. During the second trimester of pregnancy a small sample of amniotic fluid is removed via a hollow needle guided through the mother's abdomen into the amniotic sac. Cells from this fluid are grown in tissue culture for four to five weeks until enough of them are present for chromosome study. Should the foetus have some detectable genetic chromosome abnormality or be of 'undesired sex', abortion is possible.

Is this method *actually* used to detect sex and then abort the unwanted sex? Officially in this country the American College of Obstetrics and Gynecology does not approve of the use of amniocentesis for sex selection; couples here must find willing doctors. (Possibly patient choice and women's control over their bodies should extend to this choice, rather than having physicians decide.) However, physicians from India, after studying in the USA, have brought this technology back home. Doctors Prithipal and Kanan Bhandari in Amritsar, Punjab, in north India set up a billboard advertising their hospital: ' . . . know the sex of your unborn child . . . with the aid of latest imported . . . equipment and sophisticated scientific techniques'. Once the Punjab authorities found out that the imported method was being used to detect and abort girls, the procedure was forbidden; but apparently the practice still continues (Chacko 1982; Roggenkamp 1984; and Kishwar in this collection).

Even though amniocentesis with subsequent cell culture provides reliable sex detection, searches for other techniques of sex detection continue around the world. Simpler, less expensive methods that use lower technology and do not require highly skilled laboratory technicians are being sought; methods that can detect sex in the first trimester to permit a safer, early abortion are also being sought.

We shall divide *these* investigations into, first, those for detecting the sex of an *embryo* (the conceptus during the first two months of gestation) and, second, those for detecting the sex of the *foetus* (after the first two months).

Embryo sex detection

Imagine a scenario in which a clinician checks the sex of a few cells from an *in vitro* fertilized (IVF) embryo (the so-called test-tube baby), and then implants the remaining cells only when they are of the wanted sex. (In mammals a whole animal can usually be formed even if a few of the early divided cells are taken away.) A removed cell could be stained for an F-body or used to prepare a karyotype. In rabbits,

Gardner and Edwards (1968) have used cells from a later stage (the blastocyst) to predict sex correctly in the 20 per cent of the embryos that were successfully implanted into rabbit does. (By the way, if a reliable sperm separation technique gets developed, *separated* sperm could be used to fertilize the eggs removed for IVF.)

A second method speculated for use in the IVF scenario is to determine whether the embryo will react to an antibody against a product of the Y-chromosome, either the HY- or the SDM-antigen. This hypothetical method would select for girls: a male embryo would clump with the antibody and could not be implanted; the female one would not react with the antibody and could be implanted (Chapman 1982).

Such methods are only proposed at the moment; furthermore, they require teams of high technology embryologists, endocrinologists, and physicians. Some simpler methods to check the sex of an embryo conceived in the usual way are currently exciting attention in the medical literature in the United States, in Great Britain, and in China.

During the second month of gestation some cells from the embryo's portion of the placenta slough off and can be found in the lower, endocervical, part of the uterus. These can be aspirated through the cervix and stained to look for F-bodies; or another stain can be used to identify the 'Barr body', a tightly wound X-chromosome found only in cells from females. In China, this Anshan aspiration technique, reported in 1975, proved to be 93 per cent accurate. Furthermore, of thirty abortions planned after the sex detection, twenty-nine were girls (Tietung Hospital 1975).

In Scotland, an elegant refinement of this method has been developed, a method that uses new recombinant-DNA biotechnologies. Through the cervix a tiny portion of the chorionic part of the placenta can be removed (biopsied). The cells removed are tested with specific DNA probes. In Scotland the probe for Y-chromosome DNA was used, with 100 per cent accurate sex prediction reported (Gosden *et al.* 1982). This biopsy technique using specific DNA probes for certain serious genetic diseases has recently intrigued several leading clinical geneticists in the USA and was just reported by a team of French physicians in the *New England Journal of Medicine* (Cowart 1983; Goossens *et al.* 1983).

Another first-trimester method that is being explored is the detection of testosterone in maternal blood. The testis of a male embryo produces androgenic hormones, such as testosterone, which cross the placenta and add to the hormones in the mother's blood. But the mother also produces androgens, and all hormone production is cyclic; to date, such measurements seem no more predictive than guessing (Glass and Klein 1981).

Foetal sex detection

In several European clinics investigators attempt to detect sex *after* the first two months by checking for testosterone in the mother's *saliva*. Foetal hormones that pass into the mother's blood also enter her saliva. But 'spit tests' reported from Austria, Switzerland, and Germany are again no more predictive than guessing (Held *et al.* 1981; Loewit *et al.* 1982).

Also, *cells* from the foetus can cross the placenta; in a second method for foetal sex detection, clinicians check maternal blood samples with fluorescence-activated cell sorters. Reports on such attempts come from Finland, Belgium, and the USA (Herzenberg *et al.* 1979; Kirsch-Volders *et al.* 1980). The results are equivocal.

After amniocentesis, clinicians would prefer a speedier method of sex detection than the four or so weeks necessary for karyotyping. A third method under investigation is *hormone level in amniotic fluid* removed by amniocentesis and measured within one day. Méan *et al.* (1981) of Switzerland found a wide range of testosterone levels, with a statistically significant difference between the *averages* from fluid surrounding male and female foetuses. However, they found so much overlap in hormone level that in 30 per cent of the cases sex could not be determined.

A fourth late-pregnancy method, *ultrasonic viewing* of penis or vulva, has been reported from at least three continents. For example, in a report from Australia, these body parts were 'seen' in 66 per cent of 137 foetuses scanned at twenty-four to forty weeks, with only a 2 per cent error (deCrespigny and Robinson 1981). In Sweden, diagnoses could be made in 74 per cent of 101 foetuses at thirty-two weeks, with 3 per cent error (Weldner 1981).

Motivations for this work

Why are so many medical scientists in so many laboratories around the world working on so many different ways to select or detect sex of the unborn? Let us suggest at least six motivations. First there is always the challenge in understanding any of nature's mysteries. Something can be known that no human beings ever knew before! Men are especially interested in solving and appropriating the mysteries that belong to women.

Second, since knowledge is said to be power, that power can be wielded. Western humankind seems to assume that nature is poorly designed and must be 'improved' by technology, that natural processes can and must be controlled.

Third is the western love affair with technology, the compulsion to make devices to control nature.

Fourth is the wish to specify the sex of one's children, a modern and an ancient wish. The difference is that now science and technology might 'grant' that wish. If we think family-planning is a good thing, why not sex-planning? Is not this reproductive freedom?

The fifth reason commonly appears in the medical literature. When a mother carries the gene for a debilitating sex-linked disease, a sex-choice technology could prevent the production of children of the sex at risk, usually male; these children would be spared a life of suffering. (Selecting against a male in such a case, however, is not the same as choosing *for* a girl.)

The sixth reason we need to examine carefully. Sex selection has been proposed as a means to control the population explosion. Let me quote from John Postgate, a British microbiologist, writing in 1973:

> The only really important problem facing humanity to-day is overpopulation. ... Multiplication in under-developed unenlightened communities is favoured, and these are the ones most prone to perpetuate the population explosion in ignorance. ... My ... panacea, one which would take advantage of such ignorance and short-sightedness ... is a pill, or other readily administered treatment which, taken at coitus, would ensure (with ... greater than 90% certainty) that the offspring would be male. ... Countless millions of people would leap at the opportunity to breed male: no compulsion or even propaganda would be needed to encourage its use. (Postgate 1973: pp. 12, 14)

Also advocating the man-child pill, Clare Booth Luce (1978) has stated:

> The determining factor in the growth of all animal populations is ... the birth rate of female offspring. Only women have babies. And only girl babies

grow up to be women. . . . In the overpopulated countries, the preference for males amounts to an obsession. . . . A pill . . . which . . . would assure the birth of a son would come as man-ah! [sic] from Heaven. (Luce 1978: pp. C–1)

Sex preferences and imbalances

Luce is accurate about the preference for males. Son preference is a reality in both developed and developing nations. In many religions sons have specific ceremonial roles. In India and in parts of Europe the dowry that must be provided with each daughter upon marriage places a burden on families. In many countries over the globe, a woman's status and her treatment by those around her are determined by the number of sons she has produced. The need to bear a son in order to have worth as a person causes us to devalue ourselves.

And in most countries we find also the desire that the *firstborn* be male. However, a burden is laid upon children who are wanted to fulfil a gender-role image in their parents' minds. Their being chosen by a technology could make them 'feel subtly harmed, controlled, or invidiously different from other children not so conceived' (Fletcher 1983: p. 248). Sons, especially chosen sons, may be driven – by others' ambitions – to succeed in materialistic ways. Roberta Steinbacher has said:

When we add to the well-documented literature on son preference the findings on firstborns and firstborn male preference, the information is devastating to women. . . . That firstborns have distinct advantages over later borns has been well-documented for years. . . . The *de facto* second class status of women in the world would be confirmed *in fact, by choice*. (Steinbacher 1983)

Certainly we all believe that all children should know that they are wanted members of their families, that girls *should* be wanted. But, the benefits that accrue to being wanted may be outweighed by the knowledge that they were 'planned-to-be-second'.

What would social relations be like if sex choice were freely available? Several conjectures and flights of the imagination have been published. Advocate Postgate's speculations are surprisingly negative:

All sorts of taboos would be expected and it is probable that a form of *purdah* would become necessary. Women's right to work . . . would probably be forgotten transiently. . . . Some might treat their women as queen ants, others as rewards for the most outstanding (or most determined) males. (Postgate 1973: p. 16)

Guttentag and Secord (1983) have studied several *actual* modern and historical populations with sex ratio imbalances. They observed that most societies with a preponderance of males have the following characteristics:

bride-price and bride-service, great importance attached to virginity, emphasis on the sanctity of the family . . . proscriptions against adultery . . . marriage at an early age, and . . . women . . . regarded as inferior to men . . . [in] reasoned judgment, scholarship and political affairs. (Guttentag and Secord 1983: p. 79)

In some such societies women are treated as possessions to be bought and sold. Paradoxically, certain countries where women are the minority so devalue the gender that they contribute further to the scarcity of females by female infanticide, girl child neglect, and bride murders.

A feminist analysis

The real heart of the problem is that sex choice technologies would nurture patriarchy. All current forms of government are patriarchal: they foster competitiveness and have hierarchies of power and privilege; 'masculine' traits, such as aggressiveness, are rewarded. 'Feminine' qualities, such as compassion and co-operation, are disparaged. The earth, seen as feminine, is exploited. (The term 'patriarchal' does not necessarily mean 'male'; there are patriarchal women, and non-patriarchal men.) We believe that this patriarchal attitude towards the living and non-living earth, the weak, the poor, the 'others', is at the root of all the problems that are threatening the very existence of human life on this planet: poverty, pollution, nuclear war, and, yes, over-population.

If we were to use sex choice technologies and use them to select for males, we would nourish and confirm this omnipresent bias for the 'masculine'. And the mushrooming patriarchy could well lead to the end of human existence.

And why choose? Tabitha Powledge has said:

[To] choose the sexes of our children . . . is one of the most stupendously sexist acts in which it is possible to engage. It is the original sexist sin . . . [Both pre- and postconception technologies] make the most basic judgment about the worth of a human being rest first and foremost on its sex. (Powledge 1981: p. 196)

Even if people were to choose girls instead of boys, they would be emphasizing patriarchal values of rank-ordering and judgementalism. Many troubles result from needless dualisms and unnecessary choices. Hoskins (1983) concludes: 'In the case of sex preselection, a reasonable stance would be *not* to choose a girl or boy, but to welcome each *child.*'

But, what about reproductive freedom? This question poses a real dilemma to the feminist. If we should advocate restrictions of research into sex choice technologies, or if we should advocate regulations against the use of such technologies, we then can be understood as suggesting to policy makers that governments ought to regulate human reproduction. Hard-won reproductive freedoms would then be jeopardized. Thus, while standing in strong opposition to these technologies, we cannot urge laws against them (Powledge 1981).

And what about the severe population problem in the world? Some say that a bit of sexist prejudice is a less grave evil than the death by starvation of large numbers of people. However, to propose sex selection for population control is to be racist and classist as well as sexist. Advocates express no interest in having the rich white minority sacrifice any of its affluence for the benefit of the poor majority. Always it is the Third World or the poor who should have fewer, or only male, children. No one acknowledges that a rich child will consume a disproportionately large share of the world's resources, by using fossil fuels from underdeveloped nations and by eating luxury foods grown by starving people. Indeed male-choice-population-control might well stabilize the present rich-white/poor-non-white gap.

The faulty ethic of such population control is that the end is used to justify the means. The end is that *Homo sapiens* must be kept going, no matter how horrible a creature 'he' becomes in planning for 'his' survival.

As a matter of fact, positive, morally good policies have been shown to lead to population reduction. Data on factors influencing the birthrate clearly demonstrate that increases in income levels, health care, employment opportunities, education, and the status of women all contribute to decreasing population growth. 'The more education women have, the fewer children they bear' (Newland 1979: p. 42).

'The countries in which [birth-rates have dropped sharply] ... are those in which the broadest spectrum of the population has shared in the economic and social benefits of significant national progress' (Rich 1973: p. 2). When no improvement is made in providing the necessities of life, family-planning programmes meet with little success.

Conclusion

Sex selection can be touted as a 'choice' for women. However, so many of the choices that women face remain within the patriarchal framework. It is hard to choose out of that framework, and hard to raise a son or a daughter less stereotypically. There may be short-term benefits in a desired family configuration, but the long-term consequences are grim if patriarchal thinking is reinforced at the moment of conceiving a new human being.

In sum, then, our first purpose is to alert women about the widespread, international, clinical interest in developing sex choice technologies. At present the only perfected technique is amniocentesis followed by selective abortion late in the second trimester, but breakthroughs in other technologies are likely to come soon.

Our second purpose is to show women that sex choice can be another way of oppressing women. Under the guise of choice we may indeed exacerbate our own oppression.

Our third purpose is to emphasize that developers of such technologies may have racist and classist (as well as sexist) motivations, whether or not obscured by their professed concern about runaway population growth.

Acknowledgements

HBH was supported in this research by the National Science Foundation (Grant no. ISP82–09516) and the National Endowment for the Humanities. The authors' views do not necessarily reflect those of NSF or NEH.

HBH was assisted and stimulated by discussions with Spelman College students and staff. We are grateful for comments on previous versions of the manuscript by Diana Axelsen, Francis Holmes, Jodi Simpson, and Roberta Steinbacher. We remain responsible, however, for the positions taken, interpretations, and any errors.

Recommended readings

Bennett, Neil G.(ed.), *Sex Selection Of Children* (New York: Academic Press 1983). A recent interdisciplinary anthology, edited by a demographer.

Hoskins, Betty B., and Holmes, Helen B., 'Technology and prenatal femicide', in Arditti, Rita, Duelli Klein, Renate and Minden, Shelley (eds), *Test-Tube Women: What Future for Motherhood?* (London and Boston: Pandora Press 1984). A feminist, biological, values, and political analysis.

Pogrebin, Letty Cottin, 'Bias before birth', chapter 5 in *Growing Up Free: Raising Your Child in the 80's* (New York: Bantam Books 1981), pp.81–101. A feminist analysis of son preference.

Raymond, Janice (section ed.), 'Sex preselection', in Holmes, Helen B., Hoskins, Betty B., and Gross, M. (eds), *The Custom-Made Child? Women-Centered Perspectives* (Clifton, NJ: The Humana Press 1981), pp. 177–224. Nine feminist essays, the first collection on this topic.

Williamson, Nancy E., *Boys or Girls? Parents' Preferences and Sex Control* Population Bulletin (Population Reference Bureau, Washington, DC 1973).

Williamson, Nancy E., 'Sex preferences, sex control, and the status of women', *Signs: Journal of Women in Culture and Society* (1976), 1:847–62. Very competent and thorough surveys and sociological analyses of the pre-1976 literature.

References

Adimoelja, A., Hariadi, R., Amitaba, I. G. B., Adisetya, P., and Soeharno, 'The separation of X- and Y-spermatozoa with regard to the possible clinical application by means of artificial insemination', *andrologia*, **9** (3) (1977), pp. 289–92.

Beernink, F. J., and Ericsson R. J., 'Male sex preselection through sperm isolation', *Fertility and Sterility*, **38** (4) (1982), pp. 493–5.

Chacko, Arun, 'Too many daughters? India's drastic cure', *World Paper* (November 1982), pp. 8–9.

Chapman, Verne M., 'Gene products of sex chromosomes', in Amann, Rupert P. and Seidel, George E., Jr. (eds), *Prospects for Sexing Mammalian Sperm* (Boulder, Co: Colorado Associated University Press 1982), pp. 115–17.

Cowart, Virginia, 'First-trimester prenatal diagnostic method becoming available in U.S.', *Journal of the American Medical Association*, **250** (10) (1983), pp. 1249–50.

Debrovner, Charles H., Foreword, in Langendoen, Sally, and Proctor, William, *The Preconception Gender Diet* (New York: M. Evans & Co. 1982), pp. 5–8.

deCrespigny, Lachlan Ch., and Robinson, Hugh P., 'Determination of fetal sex with ultrasound', *Medical Journal of Australia*, **2** (25 July 1981), pp. 98–100.

Ericsson, Ronald J., 'Isolation and storage of progressively motile human sperm', *andrologia*, **9** (1) (1977), 111–14.

Ericsson, Ronald J., and Glass, Robert H., 'Functional differences between sperm bearing the X- or Y-chromosome', in Amann, Rupert P., and Seidel, George E., Jr. (eds), *Prospects for Sexing Mammalian Sperm* (Boulder, Co: Colorado Associated University Press 1982), pp. 201–11.

Fletcher, John C., 'Ethics and public policy: Should sex choice be discouraged?', in Bennett, Neil G. (ed.), *Sex Selection of Children* (New York: Academic 1983), pp. 213–52.

Gardner, R. L., and Edwards, R. G., 'Control of the sex ratio at full term in the rabbit by transferring sexed blastocysts', *Nature*, **218** (1968), pp. 346–8.

Glass, Allan R., and Klein, Thomas, 'Changes in maternal serum total and free androgen levels in early pregnancy: Lack of correlation with fetal sex', *American Journal of Obstetrics and Gynecology*, **140** (1981), pp. 656–60.

Goossens, Michel, Dumez, Yves, Kaplan, Liliana, Lupker, Mieke, Chabret, Claude, Henrion, Roger, and Rosa, Jean, 'Prenatal diagnosis of sickle-cell anemia in the first trimester of pregnancy', *New England Journal of Medicine*, **309** (14) (1983), pp. 831–3.

Gosden, J. R., Mitchell, A. R., Gosden, C. M., Rodeck, C. H., and Morsman, J. M, 'Direct vision chorion biopsy and chromosome-specific DNA probes for determination of fetal sex in first-trimester prenatal diagnosis', *The Lancet*, **2** (25 December 1982), pp. 1416–19.

Guerrero, Rodigo, 'Association of the type and time of insemination within the menstrual cycle with the human sex ratio at birth', *New England Journal of Medicine*, **291** (20) (1974), pp. 1056–9.

Guttentag, Marcia, and Secord, Paul F., *Too Many Women? The Sex Ratio Question* (Beverly Hills: Sage Publications 1983).

Harlap, Susan, 'Gender of infants conceived on different days of the menstrual cycle', *New England Journal of Medicine*, **300** (26) (1979), pp. 1445–8.

Held, K. R., Burck, U., and Koske-Westphal, Th., 'Pränatale geschlectsbestimmung durch den GBN-speicheltest. Ein vergleich mit den Ergebnissen der pränatalen chromosomendiagnostik', *Geburtshilfe und Frauenheilkunde*, **41** (1981), pp. 619–21.

Herzenberg, L. A., Bianchi, D. W., Schröder, J., Conn, H. M., and Iverson, G. M., 'Fetal cells in the blood of pregnant women: detection and enrichment by fluorescence-activated cell sorting', '*Proceedings of the National Academy of Science* (USA), **76** (1979), pp. 1453–5.

Hoskins, Betty B. 'When not to choose: A case study', paper presented at An Association of Liberal Religious Scholars Collegium, October, Craigville, Massachusetts.

Kirsch-Volders, M., Lissens-Van Assche, E., and Susanne, C., 'Increase in the amount of fetal lymphocytes in maternal blood during pregnancy', *Journal of Medical Genetics*, **17** (1980), pp. 267–72.

Langendoen, Sally, and Proctor, William, *The Preconception Gender Diet* (New York: M. Evans & Co. 1982).

Loewit, von K., Kraft, H. G., and Brabec, W., 'Zur geschlechtsbestimmung des fetus aus dem speichel der mutter', *Wiener klinische Wochenschrift*, **94** (8) (16 April 1982), pp. 223–6.

Lorrain, J., and Gagnon, R., 'Sélection préconceptionelle du sexe', *L'Union Médicale du Canada*, **104** (1975), pp. 800–3.

Luce, Clare Booth, 'Next: Pills to make most babies male', *Washington Star* (19 July 1978), C–1, C–4.

Méan, M., Pescia, G., Vajda, D., Pelber, J. B., and Magrini, G., 'Amniotic fluid testosterone in prenatal sex determination', *Journal de Génétique humaine*, **29** (4) (1981), pp. 441–7.

Newland, Kathleen, *The Sisterhood of Man* (New York: W. W. Norton 1979).

Postgate, John, 'Bat's chance in hell', *New Scientist*, **58** (841) (1973), pp. 12–16.

Powledge, Tabitha, 'Unnatural selection: On choosing children's sex', in Holmes, Helen B., Hoskins, Betty B., and Gross, M. (eds), *The Custom-Made Child? Women-Centered Perspectives* (Clifton, NJ: The Humana Press 1981), pp. 193–9.

Rich, William, *Smaller Families Through Economic and Social Progress*, Monograph 7 (Washington, DC: Overseas Development Council 1973).

Roggenkamp, Viola, 'Abortion of a special kind. Male sex selection in India', in Arditti, Rita, Duelli Klein, Renate, and Minden, Shelley (eds), *Test-Tube Women. What Future for Motherhood?* (London and Boston: Pandora Press 1984).

Steeno, O., Adimoelja, A., and Steeno, J., 'Separation of X- and Y-bearing human spermatozoa with the Sephadex gel-filtration method', *andrologia*, **7** (1975), pp. 95–7.

Steinbacher, Roberta, 'Sex preselection: From here to fraternity', in Gould, Carol (ed.), *Beyond Domination: New Perspectives on Women and Philosophy* (Totowa, NJ: Rowman and Allenheld 1983).

Stolkowski, J., and Choukroun, J., 'Preconception selection of sex in man', *Israel Journal of Medical Sciences*, **17** (1981), pp. 1061–6.

Stolkowski, J., and Duc, M., 'Rapports ioniques: (K^+/Ca^{2+} + Mg^{2+}) et (K^+ + Na^+/Ca^{2+} +Mg^{2+}) dans l'alimentation de femmes n'ayant que des enfants du même sexe. Enquête rétrospective', *L'Union Médicale du Canada*, **106** (1977), pp. 1351–5.

Tietung Hospital, 'Fetal sex prediction by sex chromatin of chorionic villi cells during early pregnancy', *Chinese Medical Journal*, **1** (1975), p. 117.

Weldner, E-M., 'Accuracy of fetal sex determination by ultrasound', *Acta Obstetricia et Gynecologia Scandinavica*, **60** (1981), pp. 333–4.

2 The continuing deficit of women in India and the impact of amniocentesis

Madhu Kishwar

I am going to focus on the use of amniocentesis in the context of an already existing deficit of women in the population of India. This chapter does not concern itself with the health risks inherent in the application of amniocentesis. It is a description of how and why amniocentesis is beginning to be used in India systematically to reduce the number of female children being born.

I would like to begin by reporting on two instances of deaths of women in Delhi in December 1983. In one case, a young woman who had been married for about fifteen months, took her own life soon after the birth of her first child – a daughter. Even before the child was born, the young woman's husband and in-laws had told her that she would not be allowed to return to her marital home if she gave birth to a daughter. Therefore, from the hospital, the woman was forced to go to her parents' house. This is considered a big social disgrace for a woman. She was so demoralized at being abandoned in this way that, fifteen days after her daughter's birth, she killed herself by dousing herself with kerosene and setting herself on fire in her parents' home.

In the same month, another case was reported in Delhi newspapers. A young woman in her early twenties gave birth in a private nursing home to her second child, another girl. On the day the baby was born, she strangled it to death, and was arrested for murder. It was suspected that she murdered her baby daughter because she feared she would be abandoned by her husband's family for failing to produce a son. These are two extreme examples of the potential consequences for women of giving birth to daughters instead of sons. Though this is not an everyday response to the birth of daughters, most families do feel bad when a girl is born. The acute preference for sons and viewing the birth of daughters as a curse has a long history in India.

India has recorded substantially fewer females than males in the population ever since the first modern census was taken in 1872. This disparity is indicated in the sex ratio defined as the number of females in the population per thousand males. From the earliest reports, the census takers were quite puzzled at the very imbalanced sex ratio in certain parts of the country.

In the beginning, they thought that it was perhaps due to under-reporting of females because of their seclusion, especially since only men were entrusted with the job of collecting census data. But slowly they began to acknowledge that, if fewer women were reported in each of the censuses, it was indeed true that there were fewer women in existence. More careful investigation in certain areas which showed especially dramatic population differences between the sexes showed that in some instances, the low sex ratio of women was, among other things, related to female infanticide. It was also found that the deficit of females was larger over much of the north-western plains. In the south and most of north-eastern India, there were, at that time, no such deficits of female population.

When the British administrators in the middle and latter parts of the nineteenth century tried to identify areas which were more prone to female infanticide, they found that it was not uniformly practised, but was mainly confined to certain landowning middle and upper castes in various parts of north-west India. With time, efforts were made to suppress the practice. Infanticide was made a collective offence punishable with collective fines imposed on each village where the sex ratio indicated a very high deficit of females, the so-called 'blood red villages'. The imposition of collective fines had a quick effect. They created a powerful incentive for the whole dominant caste group in the village and not just particular families to protect female infants. As a result, female infanticide began to diminish.

However, this governmental measure seems to have had an impact only on the most blatant forms of violence. Those areas and caste groups which till then had the most dramatic imbalances in the sex ratio began to register improvement in female survival chances. Government intervention seems to have left untouched the more widely prevalent practice of fatal forms of neglect of female children. This is borne out by the all India census figures during the last century. The 1901 census recorded 972 females per 1000 males. By 1981, the figure had declined to 935 females per 1000 males. The total deficit in the female population grew from 3 million in 1901 to more than 22 million in 1981.

This form of neglect involves a very systematic discrimination in food allocation and other necessities for survival. A key point is that this discrimination in food allocation does not only take place in situations of absolute scarcity. It is not as if the family discriminates only in circumstances of acute poverty. In fact, boys get relatively far more preferential treatment and better survival chances than do girls among castes and communities which are relatively better off.

Another very important area of neglect is health care. In situations where infant diarrhoea is so prevalent and contributes to more than 80 per cent of infant deaths in the country, all you have to do is neglect the child for two or three days if it has diarrhoea or some other such ailment and the child is finished. Discriminatory neglect of girl children is also reflected in hospital admission figures. Even though girls tend to suffer more from nutritional deficiencies and therefore are in greater need of health care, the all India overall admission rate to hospitals shows that parents are far more reluctant to take baby girls for medical care when they are sick. It has been found that in most children's wards, for approximately every two baby boys admitted, only one baby girl is admitted. This all India figure was illustrated by a small survey we conducted in some Delhi hospitals. This imbalance is reflected not just in the admission rate. Girls are also likely to be brought to hospital at a much later stage of illness, when they are nearly dying, so that the mortality rate, even among those few female children who are brought to hospitals, is much higher in comparison to that of boys. There are other small studies which report an overall mortality rate among baby girls in many parts of India as about 50 per cent higher than that for baby boys. This discriminatory fatality rate is essentially due to a systematic neglect of baby girls to the point of letting them die. In this context, I would like to mention a recent study done in West Bengal. The study focused on two villages, one in which land reforms have been fairly successful and one in which efforts at land reform were not successful, simply because there was not enough land to go around. The village, Kuchni village, that has undergone fairly successful land reform has a much lower proportion of landless poor families. Only 18 per cent of sample children from

Kuchni village were from landless poor families, compared to 60 per cent of children from the other villages. However, even though the village which has a very poor record of land reforms does, as expected, show a much higher overall rate of malnutrition, the relative rate of undernutrition of girls was much higher than that of boys in the village which had experienced land reforms and greater prosperity, and which had an overall lower rate of undernutrition. In other words, almost all of the benefits of economic prosperity, including better nutrition and health care went to male children. Female children stayed more or less at the level at which they were before the land reforms. Thus the relative discrimination was much less in a village that was economically worse off. If you understand this aspect of discrimination, you see that progress and economic development and many other things can have very differential impacts on women's and men's lives, and sometimes can even have a harmful impact on women's lives.

There is evidence, for instance, that as the family makes the transition from being among the landless poor to becoming small peasant proprietors, land rights almost always tend to be bestowed on the male head or whoever the government sees as the male head of the family, and thus the relative status of women is downgraded. A landless poor woman, working on a par with her husband, is seen as an equal wage earner, but once she becomes the wife of a small holding peasant, she is seen as a dependent and is therefore downgraded.

In this overall context, discrimination and neglect of baby girls is being emulated by castes and communities among whom there was no such tradition previously. This may help explain why the overall deficit has grown from 972 females per 1000 males to 935 per 1000 in the course of this century. It must, therefore, be seen as a modern phenomenon, and not just as a hangover of a traditional past. It is in this context that the coming of a technology for antenatal sex determination tests assumes very fearful dimensions.

So far there has been no systematic reporting on this issue. What I say now, therefore, is primarily a collection of impressions of those few who have been monitoring the growth of the use of amniocentesis in several parts of India. The spread of this technology and the opening of 'clinics' for this purpose started in relatively prosperous areas such as Punjab, Haryana and western Maharashtra. All these areas have undergone tremendous advances in agricultural production and are dominated by rich peasant castes. It is from these areas that the sex determination tests are spreading to other areas and are proliferating at ferocious speed. It is not just confined to urban centres where most innovations take off. I have seen such clinics in various villages and small towns in certain parts of the country.

Whatever other potential advantages sex determination tests may have, they are likely to be used in India as an incentive to destroy female foetuses. This is borne out by the few instances of data gathering in this country. For instance, when the All India Institute of Medical Sciences, at New Delhi, introduced these tests about six years ago, ostensibly to discern genetic disorders, they found that seven out of eight parents who came for the test did so with the specific purpose of aborting in case the foetus was found to be female. The Institute was flooded with requests for abortions in cases where the woman was found to be carrying a female foetus. Some of the clinics that have mushroomed over the last two or three years perform the tests relatively inexpensively, almost on a mass production basis. They proclaim very loudly that the birth of sons is the primary purpose of these tests. They do not make any bones about it. They advertise through leaflets, newspapers and magazines: 'Come for this test so that you don't have an unwanted daughter born to you.'

And so we are left with the question of what to do, knowing full well what is in store. What answers have been proposed thus far? The most common demand has been that the government should impose a ban on these tests. But I personally feel quite hesitant in demanding a government ban, because we know from experience that all it usually does is send a practice underground, thus making the practice more hazardous for the woman's health. It does not really solve the problem. For instance, just as violent forms of female infanticide turned into fatal neglect and did not improve the overall survival rate of women, there is no proof that if a girl is born she has a better chance of surviving in a family that has already determined that they do not want a daughter. This also ties up with another question: if we accept that abortion should be legal, how can we say that killing female foetuses should be illegal? In some cases, there may be no visible pressure on the woman to discriminate against her own female children. If in some situations, the woman or the family voluntarily opt for female foeticide, do we really have a right to stop them? Besides the complex moral issues involved, we are dealing with basic questions about why, in a given culture at a particular time, the life of females is so devalued that even when a woman is contributing in very important ways as the economic mainstay of the family, she is easily dispensable. What is it that makes her so?

It seems that this culture of devaluation of female lives is rooted in a situation of the near total economic and political disinheritance of women. This has been accentuated further by various economic and political developments in the last few decades, such as changes in land tenure systems and changes in technology. For instance, in some of the green revolution areas such as Punjab, where there have been tremendous advances in agriculture, employment opportunities for women are among the lowest in India. Studies have found that in most areas, women from landless poor families do not find more than forty-five to sixty days of paid employment per year in the fields. The introduction of new technology has displaced women by the millions. For instance, hand threshing of rice and grinding of corn were traditionally women's jobs. But as soon as threshing or grinding machines come to be used, millions of women are pushed out and men take over the jobs. In other words, as soon as the job becomes less drudgery oriented, requires less physical labour and provides a better income, men come and take these jobs away from women. Women are rendered more and more peripheral to the economy. They have to eke out a living by more and more miserable means and get less and less in return for their labour.

Similarly the last several decades have seen a further consolidation of land ownership in the hands of men at the cost of women's rights. Thus while women's labour plays a crucial role on the family farm, their status is like that of bonded labour who have no control over the products of their labour or over the land on which they work. Thus they are denied basic control over their own lives, and are made to feel dependent on men for their very survival. Added to the patriarchal ownership of property is the structure of the patrilocal family which ensures the political powerlessness of women in the family, the community and the village.

It is crucially important to change this power imbalance between men and women in the family in order to resist the increasing devaluation of women's lives. It is only thus that women can acquire a say in deciding what kind of health technology should be used and for what purpose. Right now, women are under tremendous pressure to produce male heirs and not burden the family by producing more than one daughter. A woman who is dependent for her very survival on men in the family is in no position to resist the pressure. In fact, she begins to see her own interest in discriminating against her own daughters, not having daughters, or having only sons, because this somewhat enhances her status in the family. But if women have independent access to means of income as well as to political power they could resist this pressure which teaches them to devalue female lives, including their own.

The problem does not seem to offer any immediate solutions. Our strategy should be to combat the rapid spread of this technology by distributing correct information about its risks and dangers while at the same time finding long-term ways to advance women's social and economic rights.

The test has not yet developed to the point of being reliable and safe enough for an expectant mother. Especially in India, where even normal health services are of appallingly poor quality, the indiscriminate commercial use of these tests by unscrupulous doctors poses a big health hazard for women. Moreover, even in predicting the sex of the child, the tests are not consistently reliable or accurate. Among those families considering use of the clinics, we need to spread this information very widely so that they do not resort to it out of ignorance or out of misinformation. This is likely to work as a disincentive but only in the short run. However, given the demand, the health industry is likely to find improved and safer methods in a few years' time.

Our long-term strategy, therefore, has to be to fight for special incentives to be made available to families for bringing up and educating daughters. This should include universal free education as well as stipends to be given to families who send their daughters to school.

However, unless families see daughters as economic assets as they now see sons, their attitude will not change substantially. Therefore we need to ensure that the current decline in women's employment is checked and that women begin to have access to decent and more remunerative forms of employment. Since a very large majority of women have to work on family farms and are not likely to seek outside employment, the issue of effective land rights for women assumes crucial significance. In a country like India, this is an essential element in the strategy to enable them to build an independent power base for women's survival.

Bibliography

Cassen, Robert, *India: Population, Economy and Society* (New York: Holmes and Meier 1978).

Kishwar, Madhu, and Vanita, Ruth (eds), *In Search of Answers: Indian women's voices from Manushi* (London: Zed Press 1984).

Manushi – a journal about women and society, Published from: C1/202 Lajpat Nagar I, New Delhi 110024, India.

Miller, Barbara, *The Endangered Sex: Neglect of Female Children In India* (Ithaca NY: Cornell University Press 1981).

Padmanabha, P., *Provisional Population Totals*, Census of India, 1981.

Panigrahi, Lalita, *British Social Policy and Female Infanticide in India* (New Delhi: Munshi Lal Manoharlal 1976).

Report of the Committee on the Status of Women in India, 1975.

3 The reproductive brothel

Gena Corea*

Newspapers assure us that such new reproductive technologies as embryo transfer, *in vitro* fertilization and artificial insemination of breeder women (usually known as 'surrogate mothers') are merely 'therapies' which kindly physicians provide for infertile women. Of course there is more to it than that. Through the years, with widespread use of the technologies, social institutions will be restructured to reflect a new reality – tightened male control over female reproductive processes. We do not know exactly how this new reality will be expressed but, as sociologist Jalna Hanmer has observed, 'we do know that in a system characterized by power imbalance, the greater the assymetry, the greater the potential abuse of the less powerful group' (Hanmer 1984: pp. 444–5).

Andrea Dworkin has described one possible expression of the new reality: the reproductive brothel (Dworkin 1983). Current male control over woman's reproduction, she points out, is sloppy. It is the farming model applied to motherhood. This is, according to Dworkin, one of two models which describes how women are socially controlled and sexually used. Under the farming model, men plant women with their seed and then harvest the crop of babies. This is inefficient. There are too many uncontrollable elements: the woman might be infertile; she might produce a bad crop one year – a defective child; there is room for her to exert her will against the man's – to secretly insert a diaphram to avoid a pregnancy or, if she wants a child, to

* A version of this paper is published in *International Women's Studies Forum*, 8 (3) (1985).

'forget' her pill; she can find some time to organize with other women and foment rebellion; each woman lives with an individual man providing her with some room for a personal relationship. Women are not all penned together, controlled, used as reproduction commodities and nothing more.

Under the second, brothel, model, women are collected together and held, unable to come and go freely. Sold as sexual commodities to men, the women are interchangeable. They are not seen as human beings with individuality and spiritual worth. The women, Dworkin writes, sell parts of their bodies 'and they also sell acts – what they say and what they do' (p. 177). This brothel model, which reduces a woman to what she sells, is efficient. The women do not get out. They are controlled with force, degradation, drugs. (For documentation, see Barry 1979.)

With the new reproductive technologies, Dworkin observes, men will be able to apply the brothel model to reproduction: 'Women can sell reproductive capacities the same way old-time prostitutes sold sexual ones . . .' (p. 182). While sexual prostitutes sell vagina, rectum and mouth, reproductive-prostitutes will sell other body parts: wombs; ovaries; eggs.

Of course, social institutions might be restructured in a less horrifying way. But the fact that women are hated in a male-supremicist culture makes it foolish to dismiss Dworkin's vision as unthinkable.

A model for the institution Dworkin envisions already exists. Many farm animals live in what are essentially reproductive brothels. On such a farm, the animal is seen as having no individuality, no spiritual worth. She is penned in under prison-like conditions. Reproductive engineers use parts of her body. They can artificially inseminate a 'superior' cow with the sperm of a 'superior' bull, remove the embryos from her body and transfer them into 'inferior' cows who will gestate the calves. Through this procedure, they can transform so-called valuable cows 'from once-a-year calf producers to machines that can produce embryos every two months . . . ' (Brotman 1983: p. 108). They can even transfer embryos of one species into female 'hatcheries' of another species. For example, in 1981, a Holstein dairy cow at the Bronx Zoo in New York gave birth to a gaur, a member of a wild endangered species.

Reproductive engineers have these techniques available to them in applying the brothel model to animal reproduction:

Artificial insemination: the fresh or frozen sperm of a 'superior' male animal can be placed into a 'gun', the gun inserted into a rod and the rod inserted into a female animal for insemination.

Superovulation: normally animals release (ovulate) only one egg a month. Reproductive engineers want many eggs 'for efficient operation' (Murray 1978: p. 292). Increased efficiency is possible because of the 1927 discovery that hormones produced by the pituitary gland affect the ovaries. It occurred to men that they could inject such hormones into a female and force the growth and ovulation of eggs from an abnormally large number of follicles – the small sacs which enclose the eggs. This is superovulation. Hormones can and experimentally have been used to force the immature ovaries of even new-born animals to produce eggs. Superovulation of very young and very old females can extend the period of their egg-production and hence of their usefulness to brothel-management.

Estrus synchronization: in order to transfer embryos, the reproductive cycles of 'donor' and recipient cows must be in accord so that when the donor ovulates and her uterus prepares itself for the implantation of a fertilized egg, the uterus of the recipient cow is also prepared to receive an egg. This can be done naturally or hormonally.

Ova recovery: after superovulating and inseminating the females, the fertilized eggs must be retrieved. Early collection techniques involved killing the females and cutting into their oviducts. 'Slaughter of donor animals augments the consistency of [egg] recovery', researchers reported (Avery and Graham 1962: p. 220). Later, they tried to recover the eggs surgically but frequently the females were left 'problem breeders', or even sterile due to surgical damage (Elsden 1978). So men moved on to non-surgical methods. Using a two-way flow catheter, they flushed fluids into her uterus and collected those fluids, along with the eggs, in a receptacle. This is the method frequently used today.

Embryo evaluation: after recovery, men inspect the embryos under dissection microscopy, eliminating those considered unfit for transfer and ranking the acceptable ones according to quality.

Twinning: Dr S. M. Willadsen has devised a method for dividing the embryo in half, producing identical twins – two animals from just one fertilized egg. An official of the International Embryo Transfer Society told me that the advantage of twinning is 'that you double – reliably, easily, fast, cheaply – the number of embryos a valuable donor produces'. Three sets of females can be used to produce the twins: the egg donors; the primary recipients in whose bodies the divided embryos are cultured; and the secondary recipients in whose bodies the embryos come to term. The animals need not be of the same species. Cows, pigs and sheep were used in various phases of one experiment on twinning (Willadsen 1981).

Embryo transfer: sometimes reproductive engineers transfer the embryo from the donor to the recipient non-surgically, inserting a catheter through the cervix to deposit the embryo in the uterus. More often, they transfer surgically because the resulting pregnancy rates (50 to 70 per cent) are better.

Caesarean section: when the pregnant cows approach full-term, veterinarians often perform Caesarean sections on them 'since the calves are usually large and the recipients are generally heifers of smaller breeds' (Seidel 1975).

One pioneer in reproductive technology estimates that techniques for maturing and fertilizing eggs in the laboratory (*in vitro* fertilization), twinning embryos and determining their sex will have commercial application before 1986 (Seidel 1981: p. 324).

How does a female live on such a brothel-farm? The words of L. J. Taylor, export development manager for The Wall's Meat Company Ltd, give some indication: 'The breeding sow should be thought of, and treated as, a valuable piece of machinery whose function is to pump out baby pigs like a sausage machine' (Singer 1975; Mason and Singer 1980: p. 35). Peter Singer and Jim Mason, who quote these words, have described the life of the sow-machine on a factory farm. It consists of pregnancy, birth, watching her babies being taken from her to be fattened for market, and then, endlessly, a repetition of the cycle: pregnancy, birth, loss of babies, insemination.

The sow is almost continually pregnant or nursing throughout her adult life. For at least ten months of every year, she is unable to walk around. After weaning, she has at most only a few days of comparative freedom before she is placed in a pen to be, once again, serviced by a boar. When she is pregnant, she is placed in a 'gestation' building. Her stall is often little bigger than she is herself – 2 feet wide and 6 feet long. She may also be tethered by a collar around her neck. She is able to stand up and lie down but does not have enough room to turn around or to exercise at all. Except at feeding time, she lives in darkness. The lights are turned off to reduce the stress and excitement in the confinement system.

About a week before the birth, farmers move her to the 'farrowing' building where she may also be closely confined in order 'to keep her in position only to eat, drink, and keep her teats exposed to the young pigs' (Mason and Singer 1980: p. 11). In Britain and in other countries she may be placed in the 'iron maiden', a frame which prevents free movement.

As I have mentioned, many animals in a reproductive brothel, considered genetically unworthy, serve as breeders for the embryos of superior animals. This distinction between the genetically worthy and unworthy is likely to increase. Writing of one scheme to obtain large-scale genetic improvement in a herd, Dr Peter Elsden of the Animal Reproduction Laboratory at Colorado State University noted that the top 10 to 20 per cent of the herd could be superovulated and used to produce many embryos, while the bottom 90 to 80 per cent of the cows could be used as recipients for those embryos. 'Therefore, the lower two-thirds of the herd is being culled in regard to their own progeny, while the top one-third of the herd is producing four times as many progeny as normal since the average number of calves per superovulation treatment is four', he wrote.

It is easy to dismiss the fate of animals as one entirely different from that of women. However, I do not believe women and animals inhabit such vastly different categories in a male supremicist world. Over centuries in many patriarchal lands, women and animals shared a common legal status. We were chattel, or moveable, animate property. Men owned slaves, cattle, concubines, beasts of burden, wives – all chattel. To this date, some laws in the United States retain common law concepts about ownership, possession and control of marital property which reflect the notion that women are economic chattel. Woman's status as sex and reproduction chattel remains in law and in practice today in the United States, as Dworkin observes. Even now, a man's 'marital right' to rape his wife is recognized in at least thirty-seven states (Shulman 1980).

Farmers now use female animals as breeders; numerous male commentators have discussed or predicted the creation of a class of professional women breeders (Davis 1937; Westoff 1978; Scott 1981; Francoeur 1970; Kieffer 1979; Packard 1979). This would be unthinkable if women were acknowledged to have the same right to bodily integrity enjoyed by men.

With the development of the surrogate motherhood industry beginning in 1977, references to professional breeders are on the increase. (The surrogate industry is one which rents women's bodies for reproductive purposes. The woman is inseminated with the customer's sperm. She then gestates the resulting baby, births it, and, for a modest fee, turns it over to the customer.) Lawyers, physicians, legislators and ethicists write of 'institutionalizing' surrogate motherhood, of the state regulating the women, of some agency certifying and licensing the mothers (Francoeur 1970: p. 106; Keane and Breo 1981: pp. 233–67). Professional breeding could become commonplace, Attorney Russell Scott writes, if 'healthy young host mothers' were offered not only payment, but social security, educational facilities and other signs of public approval as well (Scott 1981: p. 218). 'There are certainly enough women available to form a caste of childbearers, especially if the pay was right', observes one bioethicist. He refers to an unemployed nurse who offered to bear a child for a California couple so she could take herself and her young daughter off welfare (Kieffer 1979: p. 73).

Social commentator Vance Packard suggests that surrogacy would provide young women with an undemanding career. 'It would help if the hired mother was of an easygoing nature and enjoyed pregnancy and TV-watching', he wrote. The women would no doubt be free to take on a physically undemanding extra job. (He suggests ticket selling at a cinema.) If the 'mercenary mother' were to gestate an embryo conceived with another woman's egg, the job should not require much of the surrogate 'in the way of education, family background, good looks, or even skin color. If the woman is simply to be an incubator, the price would certainly be lower than if she contributed half the baby's heredity'. In South Texas, he wrote, 'pleasant, conscientious Mexican–American girls' might leap at a fee of $5000 for bearing a child and girls (sic) south of the border might leap at half that fee. 'If lawyers can arrange Mexican divorces for Americans', wrote Packard, 'they surely can arrange Mexican gestations' (Packard 1979: pp. 268–9).

Fees paid to 'host mothers' would probably vary with the country, as several commentators have suggested. Mexican women would do it for less. When it becomes possible to transfer human embryos routinely from one woman to another (and it has already been done experimentally), then the way opens up to use Third World women to gestate babies for wealthier westerners.

The president of a US foundation which helps arrange surrogate pregnancies told me: 'If we could cross international lines, then $1000 is a significant sum of money, whereas here [in the US], it's just a week or a month's wages.' Asked what countries he had in mind, he replied: 'Central America would be fine.' It is 'inevitable' that the United States go to other parts of the world and 'rely on their support' in providing surrogate mothers, he thinks. Comparing the United States to the city and Central America to the country, he pointed out that 'the cities are always supported by the country'.

A Third World surrogate mother would not even need to be healthy. 'The mother could have a health problem which could be quite serious', he said. 'However if her diet is good and other aspects of her life are o.k., she could become a viable mother for genuine embryo transfer.'

His foundation issues a quarterly directory containing pictures of North American women willing to serve as breeders. One photograph displays Number 36, 'Gabriel', an attractive woman wearing a blouse with a low neckline. An entry describing each available woman appears in the Spring 1982 Directory. An example:

> Martha F., *Address*: Escondido, Ca. *Pregnant*: No. *Status*: Divorced. *Employer*: County . . . *Birth Date*: 6–11–48. *Height*: 5′2″. *Weight*: 110. *Hair*: Blond. *Racial Origins*: Caucasian. *Children*: Kammy, Age 14 and Crissy, Age 10. *Medical*: Normal delivery both children . . . no surgery or other problems. Medical release and detailed medical history completed. *Could begin*: Immediately. *Insurance*: Greater San Diego. *Expenses Anticipated*: $20,000. *Photographs*: Available. *Contact*: By mail forwarding. *Comments*: My oldest child is a mentally gifted child. (Interested in planned or surrogate parenting.)

Sometimes the reproductive prostitute is or was a sexual prostitute as well. In Britain a childless couple hired a 19-year-old prostitute for $5500 to bear a baby for them conceived through artificial insemination with the husband's sperm. The couple entered London's Bow Street Magistrates' Court, surveyed the women who paraded to pay their regular fines, and chose one. That women would not bear them a child but agreed, for a finder's fee of $925, to locate a prostitute who would and did (Scott 1981).

Setting up stables of surrogate mothers would be establishing a primitive form of the reproductive brothel. The assembly-line approach would be used, but only to a minor degree. ('Some of the surrogates are pregnant, some are being inseminated, some are waiting to be selected', an attorney who operates a surrogate business told me in 1982. 'About four or five are waiting to get final reports in from the physician.') With improvements in technology, a brothel employing much more sophisticated assembly-line techniques and providing greater control over women becomes possible.

As I envision it, most women in a reproductive brothel would be defined as 'non-valuable' and sterilized and, in this way, their progeny culled. This vision came to me after repeatedly seeing reproductive engineers link their new technologies – *in vitro* fertilization, embryo transfer, egg banks – with sterilization (Muller 1961; Fletcher 1974; Fletcher 1976; Seed and Seed 1978; Djerassi 1979; Edwards 1979). They invariably suggest that the sterilization will benefit those operated upon. Women could be sterilized knowing that if they later want a child, they can have one through use of the new technologies. In this way, women would be able to avoid modern steroidal contraception.

In the United States, women of colour probably would be labelled 'non-valuable', sterilized and used as breeders for the embryos of 'valuable' women. The white women judged genetically superior and selected as egg donors would be turned into machines for producing embryos. Through superovulation, 'valuable' females as young as 2 years and some as old as 50 or 60 could be induced to produce eggs.

Reproductive engineers would engage in three major activities in the brothel: 1 getting eggs; 2 manipulating them; 3 transferring embryos.

Getting eggs

There are a number of ways engineers might recover or, as they term it, 'capture' eggs from women. They could flush them out of women using the technique developed by Drs Richard and Randolph Seed with the medical team at the Harbor-UCLA Medical Center. (The Seed brothers worked on egg flushing and embryo transfer for six years in cows before moving on to women. They had their first human success in 1983 when they established pregnancies through embryo transfer in two women in Torrance, California.) However, the Seeds' flushing procedure would probably not yield the necessary quantity of eggs. It is also unlikely that engineers would use two techniques employed experimentally in animals: placing tubular instruments inside the women's reproductive tracts and keeping them there permanently so that eggs would pass into the instruments and out of the bodies; and relocating women's ovaries to make it easier to get at the eggs. These techniques had been 'found wanting' in animals and abandoned (Betteridge 1981: p. 8).

Eggs are far more likely to be obtained by extracting them directly from the ovaries, a procedure which requires control over the female cycle. In *Farm Journal* in 1976, Earl Ainsworth, identifying the factor which prevented farmers from treating sows totally as machines, wrote: 'Estrus control will open the doors to factory hog production. Control of female cycles is the missing link to the assembly-line approach' (Mason and Singer 1980: p. 19). The 'missing link' to the assembly-line, brothel approach to human reproduction is being forged in *in vitro* fertilization clinics around the world where teams are working intensively to control the cycles of women.

In the brothel, on the appropriate days of their cycles, women would line up for Pergonal shots which will stimulate their ovaries. Engineers would superovulate only the top 10 to 20 per cent of the female population in the brothel. Then, after following the development of the eggs through ultrasound and blood tests, they would operate on the women to extract the eggs. Perhaps they would allow the women to heal from the operation every other month so that women would only be subjected to surgery six times per year.

To obtain eggs, engineers could also do what they now do with certain cows. When the championship cow Sabine 2A died in 1982 during a Caesarean section, embryologists from the firm Genetic Engineering Inc. removed her ovaries, obtained thirty-six eggs from them, and froze the eggs. During her lifetime, Sabine's embryos had been fetching $10,000 or more on the embryo transfer market and when the eggs from the dead Sabine are thawed and fertilized *in vitro*, they may fetch the same (Brotman 1983). In the reproductive brothel, as a valuable woman dies, engineers could operate on her, remove her ovaries and salvage eggs from those ovaries, perhaps by using enzymes to eat away the connective tissue and release hundreds of thousands of eggs. They could then freeze the eggs for future *in vitro* fertilization and transfer into a 'non-valuable' female. A woman could be used for reproduction long after she is dead.

Not only could dead women be used in reproductive brothels. So could women who were never even born. A female embryo could be developed just to the point where an ovary emerges and then the ovary could be cultured so that engineers could get eggs from it. The full woman would never be allowed to develop. Just her ovary.

Partial ectogenesis – culturing organ rudiments from their earliest appearance to a mature state – is already well established as a technique used in certain biological studies. If various fragmented procedures reported by different scientists could be brought together and, in combination, used in one species, mature organs might soon be produced externally from a fertilized egg, embryologist Dr Clifford Grobstein has predicted. One of the organs men have extensively investigated is the ovary. By maturing the ovary externally, Grobstein wrote, a supply of eggs for *in vitro* fertilization could be provided without surgical intervention in a woman's body (Grobstein 1981: p. 48).

Manipulating eggs

Once the eggs have been recovered, reproductive engineers along the assembly line could manipulate them in a number of ways:

Twin the embryos, producing two humans out of one embryo.

Use the eggs of 'non-valuable' women for clones, destroying the egg nuclei with lasers and injecting the nuclei of valuable men.

Remove the female genetic component from the egg and inject two sperm into the egg, producing a child with two fathers and no mother.

Genetically engineer the embryo for various qualities. If ever partial or total ectogenesis were applied to humans, it would be 'no more than a game for the "manfarming biologist" to change the subject's sex, the colour of its eyes, the general proportions of body and limbs, and perhaps the facial features', wrote biologist Jean Rostand, overconfidently (Rostand 1959: p. 84).

Fertilize the eggs in the laboratory using a culture media concocted from bits and pieces of women. 'We made our culture fluids resemble the female reproductive tract by adding very small pieces of human uterus or Fallopian tube ... ' wrote *in vitro* fertilization pioneers Patrick Steptoe and R. G. Edwards (Edwards and Steptoe 1980: p. 54). Another reproductive engineer used 'minced fragments of [women's] fallopian tubal mucosa' (Shettles 1955).

Select the sex of the embryo by fertilizing the egg with either gynosperm (female-engendering) or androsperm (male-engendering).

Researchers are hard at work now trying to separate these two types of sperm. Should they fail, there is another way to predetermine the child's sex. Engineers could snip a few cells off the fertilized egg to check its gender. Most female embryos could simply be discarded. The brothel administration would decide how many would be needed.

Transferring embryos

Once the embryo has been manufactured, reproductive engineers would have several options.

They could freeze the embryo in the bank for later use. Or they could immediately transfer the embryo into a woman in the lower 80 to 90 per cent of the female population. These would be the breeders, the women who had been called 'surrogate mothers' in the early stage of the reproduction revolution when engineers had been conscious of the need for good public relations.

The transferred embryo might gestate in the breeder for the entire nine-month pregnancy. When delivery time approached, the breeder would find no cosy 'birthing rooms' in the brothel, but rather an assembly line. The description women gave of their obstetrical experiences in American hospitals in the 1950s are likely to be as apt for the brothel of the future: 'They give you drugs, whether you want them or not, strap you down like an animal' (p. 44). 'Women are herded like sheep through an obstetrical assembly line, are drugged and strapped on tables while their babies are forceps-delivered' (p. 45). 'I felt exactly like a trapped animal ...' (Shultz 1958 and 1959).

Alternatively, engineers could transfer the embryo into a breeder, allow it to gestate for a certain number of months, and then remove the foetus by Caesarean section at whatever point at which their incubators could take over. (Today that point is twenty-one-weeks gestation.) In the incubator, they would perform surgery on the foetus, inoculate it or undertake whatever alterations they deemed desirable.

The breeder into whom an embryo is placed need not be alive. This possibility is suggested by several recent cases in which the bodies of brain dead pregnant women were kept functioning until the foetus had developed enough to be delivered. In one case, a 27-year-old woman suffered a fatal seizure when she was twenty-two-weeks pregnant. Her husband and other family members wanted the woman's body kept in operation until the foetus became viable. Physicians put her on a life-support system. Their most difficult medical challenges during the nine weeks they maintained the dead woman, they report, were keeping control of the woman's many failing body functions and combating infection. The woman developed diabetes insipidus and Addison's disease and, periodically, a blood infection throughout the body. Doctors did blood studies on the dead woman every two hours. They performed a Caesarean section on her more than two months after she had been declared dead, extracted a healthy baby and then removed the life-support apparatus. She stopped breathing. Relatives reportedly expressed 'a great deal of pleasure' at the birth (*Star-Ledger* 1983).

'The experience left me with real confidence that this can be done without any great difficulties. . . . In the future, I'll suggest to family members that the option is there'. Dr Russell K. Laros Jr. of the Department of Obstetrics, Gynecology and Reproductive Sciences at the University of California School of Medicine in San Francisco, said (OGN 1983: p. 2).

(Immediately over the Newark *Star-Ledger*'s account of the birth – 'Brain Dead Woman Gives Birth' – appeared a photograph of smiling parents holding their infants, the nation's first test-tube twins.)

Perhaps in the distant future, few women, dead or alive, will be required. If reproductive engineers have developed an artificial womb, they might place the cultured embryo directly into The Mother Machine.

The reproductive brothel is one possible institution within which men might control women, or various groups of women, in the future. Other scenarios involving use of the new technologies are also conceivable. Women need to grapple with this issue. Jalna Hanmer has urgently called for: 1 a series of meetings within feminist movements around the world on what action to take; 2 an international feminist network to monitor developments in these new reproductive technologies; and 3 an International Tribunal on Medical Crimes Against Women. I add my voice, urgently, to hers.

References

Avery, T. L., and Graham, E. F., 'Investigations associated with the transplanting of bovine ova: III. Recovery and fertilization', *J. Reprod. Fertil.* (1962), pp. 212–17.

Barry, Kathleen, *Female Sexual Slavery* (Englewood Cliffs, New Jersey: Prentice-Hall Inc. 1979).

Betteridge, K. J., 'An historical look at embryo transfer', *J. Reprod. Fertil.*, **62** (1981), pp. 1–13.

Brotman, Harris, 'Engineering the birth of cattle', *New York Times Magazine* (15 May 1983).

Davis, Kingsley, 'Reproductive institutions and the pressure for population', *The Sociological Review* (1937).

Djerassi, Carl, *The Politics of Contraception* (New York; London: W. W. Norton & Co. 1979).

Dworkin, Andrea, *Right-Wing Women* (New York: Perigee Books 1983).

Edwards, R. G., 5 January 1979, Letter to US Ethics Advisory Board in *Appendix: HEW Support of Research Involving Human In Vitro Fertilization and Embryo Transfer* (4 May 1979). US Government Printing Office, Washington, D.C.

Edwards, R. G., and Steptoe, Patrick, *A Matter of Life* (New York: William Morrow and Co. Inc. 1980).

Elsden, Peter, 'Advances in embryo transfer techniques', *Holstein Friesian World* (10 February 1978).

Fletcher, Joseph, *The Ethics of Genetic Control: Ending Reproductive Roulette* (Garden City, New York: Anchor Press/Doubleday 1974)

Fletcher, Joseph, 'Ethical aspects of genetic controls', in Shannon, Thomas A. (ed.), *Bioethics* (New York/Ramsey, New Jersey: Paulist Press 1976).

Francoeur, Robert T., *Utopian Motherhood* (New York: Doubleday & Co. Inc. 1970).

Grobstein, Clifford, *From Chance to Purpose: An Appraisal of External Human Fertilization* (Reading, Mass: Addison-Wesley Publishing Co. 1981).

Hanmer, Jalna, 'A womb of one's own', in Arditti, Rita, Duelli Klein, Renate, and Minden, Shelley, (eds), *Test-Tube Women* (Boston and London: Pandora Press 1984).

Keane, Noel P., with Breo, Dennis L., *The Surrogate Mother* (New York: Everest House 1981).

Kieffer, George H., *Bioethics: A Textbook of Issues* (Reading, Mass: Addison-Wesley Publishing Co. 1979).

Mason, Jim, and Singer, Peter, *Animal Factories* (New York: Crown Publishers Inc. 1980).

Muller, Herman J., 'Human evolution by voluntary choice of germ plasma', *Science*, **134** (3480) (1961).

Murray, Finnie A., 'Embryo transfer in large domestic mammals', in

Daniel, Joseph C., Jr. (ed.), *Methods in Mammalian Reproduction* (New York; San Francisco; London: Academic Press 1978).

OGN, 'Maintenance of brain-dead gravida held viable course', *Ob. Gyn. News*, **18** (11) (1983), p. 2.

Packard, Vance, *The People Shapers* (New York: Bantam 1979).

Rostand, Jean, *Can Man Be Modified?* (New York: Basic Books 1959).

Scott, Russell, *The Body As Property* (New York: The Viking Press 1981).

Seed, Randolph W., and Seed, Richard C., Statement before the Ethics Advisory Board of the Department of Health, Education and Welfare, 13 October 1978.

Seidel, George E., Jr., 'Embryo transfer', *Charolais Bull-O-Gram* (April/May 1975).

Seidel, George E., Jr. 'Superovulation and embryo transfer in cattle', *Science*, **211** (4479) (1981), pp. 351–8.

Shettles, Landrum P., 'A morula stage of human ovum developed in vitro', *Fertility and Sterility*, **6** (4) (1955), pp. 287–9.

Schulman, Joanne, 'The marital rape exemption in the criminal law', *Clearinghouse Review*, **14** (6) (1980), pp. 538–40.

Shultz, Gladys Denny, 'Journal mothers report on cruelty in maternity wards', *Ladies Home Journal* (May 1959).

Singer, Peter, *Animal Liberation* (New York: Avon Books 1975).

Star-Ledger (Newark, NJ) 'Brain dead woman gives birth', 31 March 1983.

Westoff, Charles F., 'Some speculations on the future of marriage and fertility', *Family Planning Perspectives,* **10** (2) (1978), pp. 79–83.

Willadsen, S. M., Lenhn-Jensen, H., Fehilly, C. B., and Newcomb, R., 'The production of monozygotic twins of preselected parentage by micromanipulation of non-surgically collected cow embryos', *Theriogenology*, **15** (1) pp. 23–7.

4 Sex choice: survival and sisterhood

Roberta Steinbacher and Helen B. Holmes

'I didn't ask to be born' is one truism which remains true, especially now that we live in a 1984 frighteningly like the *1984* of George Orwell. Indeed, until a few decades ago, when 'birth control' became the relatively reliable spectrum of technologies that the phrase represents today, most of our parents could say that they did not choose to have us born either. For privileged people now, the question of whether to have a child and when is very largely a matter of choice.

But now – in 1984 fittingly – it is not only the birth of children *per se* that is the matter of choice. With the advent of sex preselection technologies, we may actually be at the dawn of an era when parents may choose which sex gets born – i.e. whether a son or a daughter will be brought into the world. The availability of that choice stems from radical developments in reproductive technology, as described by Holmes and Hoskins in this book.

Sex preferences

We have all grown up knowing that boys are preferred to girls:

> First comes love, then comes marriage,
> Then comes [name] with a baby carriage.
> I wish you love, I wish you joy,
> I wish you first a baby boy.
> And when his hair begins to curl,
> I wish you then a baby girl. (*autograph book, USA*)

Through the centuries and round the world it has been the same. Look at some examples collected by Pogrebin in 1980:

Even a deformed son is better than the brightest, most skilled girl. (*China*)

If the tenth too, is a girlchild
I will cut both of your feet off,
To the knees I'll cut your feet off,
Both your arms up to the shoulders,
Both your eyes too, I will put out,
Blind and crippled you will be then,
Pretty little wife, young woman. (*Bulgaria*)

Salut' e figli maschi (after a sneeze).
(Good health and male children.) (*Italy*)

Furthermore, the results of social science research on parental preferences for children's sex make the societal implications of sex choice staggering – truly post-Orwellian. For historically, anthropologically, sociologically, and psychologically, the choices of both men and woman have been – and remain, as most recent studies indicate – heavily weighted for male firstborn children. The Dinitz, Dynes and Clark study of 1954 reported that 62 per cent of the males and 58 per cent of the females sampled preferred firstborn sons. If they were to have only one child, then 92 per cent of the men and 66 per cent of the women chose a boy. Markle and Nam in 1971 found that 80 per cent of male respondents and 79 per cent of the females opted for a firstborn son. In 1976, summarizing forty years of cross-cultural reports and attitudinal and behavioural studies, Williamson noted no decline in son preference over that span of time in the United States, Europe, or developing countries. Very recently in a 1984 study in Texas, Pharis and Manosevitz found that 62 per cent of the students surveyed preferred a firstborn son.

On the other side of the gender ledger, meanwhile, preference for firstborn daughters has remained virtually absent (4 per cent, 12 per cent, and 6 per cent in the three studies mentioned above).

Effect of the women's movement

Did the growth of the women's movement in the United States affect these preferences? In 1974 Norman found in a sample of 152 students that only 46.9 per cent chose a firstborn son. However, a close look at his data reveals that 45.1 per cent indicated 'no preference' and therefore that only 8 per cent selected firstborn daughters. Essentially then, these results are no different from those cited above. Furthermore, when these students were also asked to choose the sex of child for a one-child family, 85.8 per cent of the males and 59 per cent of the females chose a son.

Perhaps those who actually support the women's movement will differ from those who do not support it in their preferences for sex of firstborns? That expectation was not borne out when Rent and Rent first tested the relationship between support for the movement and firstborn preference in 1977. Surveying students at two women's colleges, for example, they found that those who gave strong and active support to the movement were more likely to express 'no preference' for sex. Those women who *did* express a sex preference, however, even those who indicated 'strong support of' or 'some agreement with' the women's movement, overwhelmingly preferred sons, even when compared to those in the 'no support' category.

Faith Gilroy of Loyola College in Maryland and Steinbacher studied this issue in 1981 (published in 1983a), through a survey of 236 college undergraduates – sixty-five females and forty-five males at a private college on the East Coast, and seventy-four women and fifty-two men at a public midwestern university. There was no relationship between support of the women's movement and sex preference by females in this sample, but males who indicated 'strong support' for the movement were unanimous in indicating no preference for sex of firstborn.

Preferences of pregnant women

Less marked preferences are reported in the rather sparse literature on sex preferences of pregnant women. The original study conducted by Uddenberg, Almgren and Nilsson in Sweden in 1971, reported no statistical significance in a 46 per cent son-preference, 32 per cent daughter-preference, and 22 per cent no-preference given by eighty-one women pregnant for the first time. In 1978, Oakley's study reported 54 per cent of the pregnant women sampled preferred sons, while 22 per cent preferred daughters, and 25 per cent had no preference. Pharis and Manosevitz in 1984 surveyed couples expecting their first child (without reporting separate figures for husband and wife) and found that 25 per cent preferred a boy, 7 per cent preferred a girl, and 48 per cent had no preference.

Expressing 'no preference' during pregnancy might be explained by the results of Tedeschi and Reiss's 1981 impression management research. Women might be motivated to avoid 'cognitive dissonance', i.e., to be unwilling to express dissatisfaction with an infant of either sex when the determination had already been made.

How do attitudes towards the women's movement correlate with sex preferences of pregnant women? Two studies have examined this question. Using the 'attitude toward women' scale, Calway-Fagen, Wallston and Gabel in 1979 surveyed pregnant women and their spouses. They found that those men and women with positive attitudes towards women's liberation showed significantly less preference for males than did those with more negative attitudes towards the movement. (They did not separate their findings by the respondent's sex.) Then Gilroy and Steinbacher in 1983 surveyed 140 women pregnant for the first time, in the last three months of their pregnancy. The women were antenatal clinic patients at a suburban hospital (40); women at two inner-city hospitals (40); patients of four private gynaecologists (30); and participants in a Lamaze class (30). Overall, 59 per cent expressed 'no preference', a contrast with the 22, 25 and 48 per cent figures in the three previous studies. However, since this Gilroy/Steinbacher survey took place near the end of pregnancy, the issue of choice was no longer hypothetical. The actual presence of the lifeforce – in either birth or death situations – could be so powerful that it might wipe out previous memories about preferences.

Most significant and discrepant from earlier research, though, is this finding: of the 41 per cent who did indicate a sex preference for firstborns, 57 per cent choose to have a girl first. From the group that expressed support for the women's movement, 35 per cent of the strong advocates and 22 per cent of the moderate advocates chose a firstborn daughter. This is not a heavy margin of preference, but it constitutes the first finding – no matter what the sample involved – that does not indicate a clear preference for male firstborns.

What is the explanation of this deviation from previous research? The most optimistic is that American society is becoming less biased, and that male and female infants are both perceived as valuable and desirable. A more likely possibility is that women actually have an underlying preference for daughters, as hypothesized by Raymond in 1981, and that the Gilroy/Steinbacher research has managed to reveal this. Still another possibility is that expectant mothers today – aware of cultural striving for sexual equality – might be reluctant to verbalize a choice that appears inappropriate, i.e. to express in a survey their adherence to sexual stereotypes.

Willingness to use sex choice technologies

Only a few researchers have asked whether, if sex selection techniques were available, the respondents would use them. In the Markle and Nam 1971 report, 26 per cent of 283 Florida students said they would like to choose sex. In 1974 Westoff and Rindfuss found that 38.8 per cent of currently married women gave positive responses. In 1977 Hartley and Pietraczyk analysed 2138 responses from a random sample of students (53 per cent of them male) in classes at five different northern California colleges. They found more acceptance of the idea than the earlier workers: a majority of their respondents (65.9 per cent) 'agreed' that the technology of sex predetermination should be available to all parents, and 44.6 per cent of them would want to use such procedures themselves. Perhaps during the 1970s, when medical technologies were burgeoning and were copiously and glowingly reported by the media, people became more ready to accept such technologies. Yet, at least among college students, the underlying preferences about sex of offspring did not change.

The 1983a Gilroy/Steinbacher study also asked college students whether they would use the technology. And, the chilling results from those who indicated yes, were that 81 per cent of the women and 94 per cent of the men preferred firstborn sons. The second, 1983b, Gilroy/Steinbacher research was the first study of sex preferences in pregnant women, that at the same time assessed their support of the women's movement *and* their willingness to select their child's sex. The question they were asked was, 'If the means were available so that you could have selected the sex of your child, would you have done so?' 18.5 per cent of the respondents answered yes to this question, and among those, the choice of sex of firstborn was split equally between males and females. Therefore, the slight preference for firstborn girls which this very recent Gilroy/Steinbacher study uncovered vanishes when technology-acceptors are identified.

Death of the female?

However devalued, controlled, feared, or exploited women have been, their indispensability to the continuation of the human race has remained a stubborn fact, conceded in even the most oppressive, patriarchal societies. However, now for the first time in human history, the power is at hand to negate that indispensability. The world's female population could be reduced to a select number of wombs needed to produce eggs, if not to carry them in gestation. In 1984, at least, the uterus is still needed after *in vitro* fertilization and even for the recent development of implanting an egg from another woman's womb, an egg fertilized by a male-determining sperm.

However, the ultimate extension of the capacity to control embryonic development outside the female body is now being developed: artificial laboratory wombs.

There is, to be blunt, the possibility of femicide.

Impossible? Unthinkable? Nothing that becomes technologically possible is unthinkable. There is no atrocity too terrible for human nature to contemplate and often carry out. This has, in fact, been the case numerous times throughout history, and has been justified as necessary to fulfil the needs and 'rights' of 'superior' individuals or races. Consider that the first European immigrants to the United States immediately abrogated the property rights of the American Indians who populated that continent – then virtually extinguished the populations of those tribes, along with their 'inferior' culture. To impose the 'progress' of the white population's mores and culture was justified as morally right. Today, the few descendents of those tribes – who did not want to believe that the people they welcomed to their land would actually destroy them – are living on reservations, or as second-class citizens in a society that still doesn't really consider them Americans.

In the 1930s and 1940s, when German Nazis killed more than 5 million Jews to obtain *Lebensraum* for the 'superior' Aryan race, there were people on the way to the gas chambers who still didn't want to believe that they would be killed, or that an attempt was being made to eradicate an entire people. There is a natural reluctance to consider horror on that scale.

And remember that since the Book of Genesis, woman has been branded as 'inferior' to man. Then reconsider whether femicide is really an impossibility.

It requires a tough honesty of mind to think through the ramifications of sex preselection, because it also requires seeing through and exposing the 'double-think' indigenous to the medical patriarchy which has developed and controlled reproductive technology in virtually all its forms: birth control methods, prenatal diagnostic technologies, the foetal monitor, Caesarean sections, *in vitro* fertilization/embryo transfer, and now sex-preselection technology. All these developments have been couched in terms and rationales 'supportive' of women's profound power to reproduce by 'freeing' them from attendant trauma of pregnancy, labour, and childbirth.

Indeed, some of these developments, to varying extents, have proven beneficial to certain women. But who also bears the costs and burdens when the male-developed reproductive benefits fail? Women. It is women who have been the guinea pigs, for instance, for testing oral contraceptives and the alleged anti-abortifacient, DES. They have experienced strokes and blood clots and cancer. It is women who have been the victims through sterilization and even death after using the male-developed IUD (intrauterine device), the Dalkon Shield.

The myth that science and technology are value-free is just that: a myth. Yet, sex preselection technology has developed and is rapidly advancing, virtually unfettered by the scientific, religious, and legal cross-examination that could provide critical checks and balances.

One of the numerous new sex detection techniques described by Holmes and Hoskins in this volume has already come under critical questioning about safety. In the United States in February, a fourteen-member task force from the National Institutes of Health, after a year-long study, concluded that ultrasound screening during pregnancy should not be done routinely. Ultrasound's 'lack of risk is only assumed rather than clearly demonstrated', their report stated, citing tests indicating that ultrasound may cause cell damage or affect antenatal growth.

Why should women assume, for instance, that other sex selection/detection techniques – for example, aspiration of cells from the placenta to detect sex chromosomes – might not later prove harmful to the mother or to those foetuses (mostly male) chosen for life? Yet the question of speeding and facilitating these techniques – presented as a means to rid society of genetic defects rather than of the unwanted sex – has taken precedence over long-term testing of safety or side effects.

Patriarchal control over reproduction

Patriarchal, religious, legal, medical, and commercial institutions have long controlled women's power of reproduction. They have exercised that control through what might be termed sublimated legitimization

(Steinbacher 1984). Rarely has reproductive power been treated simply as the natural human process it actually is.

Instead religion controls it by requiring women's children to remain in a state of 'original sin' until it confers baptism – in essence, a second birth bestowed by the hands of males. Additionally, through many church doctrines, female reproductive power is: negated (holy women must be celibate); prescribed (by prohibiting 'artificial' birth control or abortion); mystified (by forbidding sex education); sanctified (by making marriage a sacrament, and childbearing a holy obligation); called unclean (purification rites required after menstruation); and often branded as a sin (through dogmatic stigma/punishment, usually only for women, for sex out of marriage, sex without procreation, or adultery) (Steinbacher 1984).

Similarly, law controls by relegating women to second-class, even 'property' status. Women's rights to inherit or hold property, exercise citizenship, or receive higher education are still denied over much of the globe. American law no longer classifies women as property, but it pronounces their children 'legitimate' or 'illegitimate' depending on the mother's state-defined relationships to males.

Right now, while lawyers are serving as paid intermediaries to arrange surrogate births, the legal profession is toying with the issue of whether the state has a compelling interest to prevent the birth of 'unhealthy' foetuses. 'Wrongful life' suits convert virtually insoluble ethical dilemmas into costly emotional and financial realities. For example, damages can be recovered on the grounds that a foetus with genetic defects was 'permitted' to be born.

While medicine obviously aids women in many ways (though usually from overall advances for human health), the profession exercises many unmerited controls over women. In reproduction particularly, medicine accomplishes these controls by representing itself as indispensable to woman's birthing process. It is also the male-dominated profession of surgery that dictates – not always from altruistic motives, and certainly not infallibly – the fate of female reproductive organs and processes. The medical profession has further prospered on reproduction through the use of multi-stage hospitalizations.

Commerce profits from medicine's monopoly over female reproduction. An obvious example is the pharmaceutical firms' monopoly on means of contraception. Consider further the costly, complex monitoring devices that are sometimes totally unnecessary. And consider the commercial supplantation of female lactation. Infant formulas that led to staggering numbers of infant deaths continue to be distributed to Third World countries.

The individuals in these patriarchal power groups will also control usage (and inevitable misusage) of sex preselection technology. Research in this area is almost entirely in the hands of males, and funded by male-controlled governmental and private agencies.

Once the process of selecting the sex of offspring can be made both convenient and inexpensive, while still producing profits, the commercial tide will not be reversible. Family planning will become simply the acting-out of what we know from the studies cited above, and from our own everyday observations. A vast majority of parents will choose to have a firstborn son. Daughters, when chosen at all, will usually be later born.

Action is needed

Those eventualities are critical for women, collectively and individually. Numerous studies clearly indicate that firstborn children are found in disproportionate numbers in positions of power and privilege. Today, even with a fifty:fifty chance of being firstborn, women are not found in those powerful, privileged positions in proportion to their numbers in society. With the higher ratio of firstborn males to firstborn females likely to result from sex preselection, women's access to social and economic power may be entirely eliminated.

Individually, when females realize that they are chosen to be second, the psychological ramifications will be incalculable. The notion of inferiority which society still dictates for women as a class, despite the women's movement, undoubtedly would be further internalized and externalized. The sharply reduced numbers of females, when they come to be 'chosen' for reproductive purposes or to be little sisters, may well be regarded (by themselves and by others) as 'chosen' for powerlessness (Fidell, Hoffman and Keith-Spiegel 1979; Steinbacher 1980; 1981; 1984).

Women, caught up now in struggling for fundamental rights for themselves and for their daughters, are ill-prepared for a future with reproductive technologies. As Zimmerman cautioned in 1981, 'For all their potential value ... [these technologies] offer ... glitter without goal and achievement. Unless women gain control of those technologies, they will find that they have created new lives for themselves today, only to have forfeited the future – an empty womb indeed.'

What can be done? It is a task that makes unprecedented demands on our collective responsibility. But apathy cannot prevail.

Moreover, a particularly finely honed caution is necessary in handling this double-edged sword – because legislation to prohibit any of these technologies would in itself be dangerous (Powledge 1981). Any regulation of human reproduction also risks cutting away women's reproductive rights.

First, women must break the protective silence surrounding sex preselection research laboratories, and boardrooms of the institutions and agencies controlling the production of these technologies. We must force the full facts and implications of this radical phenomenon into the open, to generate the sort of vigorous public debate that can set into motion critical checks and balances.

More than ever before it is up to women to raise the moral consciousness of both men and unconvinced women about the invidiousness of valuing persons on the basis of their sex alone. Then we must make them realize that sex preselection technologies are unrelated to generally accepted concepts of disease.

Finally, it is crucial to each of us to look with unblurred vision at the motives and morality of a mindset that would preselect the sex of children. We concur with Powledge in her 1981 judgement of these technologies as 'the original sexist sin . . . they make the most basic judgment about the worth of a human being rest first and foremost on its sex'. We must remember the so-often forgotten fact about human society: whenever any individual – or group of individuals – prospers or succeeds at the expense of others' well-being, the so-called winner loses his or her own worth. The use of sex selection technologies could thus make losers of us all.

Should sex selection technologies become widely available, then we must all strive to see that they are used as advances for humanity, not just as technological achievements. We must strive to see that they are used to benefit both sexes, not to damage or destroy one. Morality and technology should be able to coexist in the technological future, every human being should be able to say, from the basis of fair and equitable numbers and status: 'I did not ask to be born . . . but my parents did choose to have me'.

Me. This woman, this man, this person.

References

Calway-Fagen, N., Wallston, B. S., and Gabel, H., 'The relationship between attitudinal and behavioral measures of sex preference', *Psychology of Women Quarterly,* **4** (1979), pp. 274–80.

Dinitz, S., Dynes, R. R., and Clarke, A. C., 'Preference for male or female children: traditional or affectional?', *Marriage and Family Living,* **16** (1954), pp. 128–30.

Fidell, L., Hoffman, D., and Keith-Spiegel, P., 'Some social implications of sex-choice technology', *Psychology of Women Quarterly,* **4** (1979), pp. 232–46.

Gilroy, F., and Steinbacher, R., 'Preselection of child's sex: technological utilization and feminism', *Psychological Reports,* **53** (1983a), pp. 671–6.

Gilroy, F., and Steinbacher, R., Unpublished data (1983b).

Hartley, S. F., and Pietraczyk, L. M., 'Preselecting the sex of offspring: technologies, attitudes, and implications', *Social Biology,* **25** (2) (1979), pp. 232–46.

Markle, G. E., and Nam, C. B., 'Sex predetermination: its impact on fertility', *Social Biology,* **18** (1971), pp. 73–82.

Norman, R., 'Sex differences in preferences for sex of children: a replication after 20 years', *Journal of Psychology,* **88** (1974), pp. 229–39.

Oakley, A., 'What makes girls differ from boys?', *New Society* (21 December 1978), pp. xii-xiv.

Pebley, A. R., and Westoff, C. F., 'Women's sex preferences in the United States: 1970 to 1975', *Demography,* **19** (1982), pp. 177–89.

Pharis, M. E., and Manosevitz, M., 'Sexual stereotyping of infants: implications for social work practice', *Social Work Research and Abstracts,* **20** (1984), pp. 7–12.

Pogrebin, L. C., 'Bias before birth', chapter 5 in *Growing Up Free: Raising Your Child in the 80's* (New York: Bantam Books 1981), pp. 81–101.

Powledge, R., 'Unnatural selection: on choosing children's sex', in Holmes, H. B., Hoskins, B. B., and Gross, M. (eds), *The Custom-Made Child? Women-Centered Perspectives* (Clifton, NJ: The Humana Press 1981), pp. 193–9.

Raymond, J., 'Sex preselection: a response', in Holmes, H. B., Hoskins, B. B., and Gross, M. (eds), *The Custom-Made Child? Women-Centered Perspectives* (Clifton, NJ: The Humana Press 1981), pp. 209–12.

Rent, C. S., and Rent, G. S., 'More on offspring sex-preference: a comment on Nancy E. Williamson's "Sex preference, sex control, and the status of women"', *Signs: Journal of Women in Culture and Society*, **3** (1977), pp. 505–15.

Steinbacher, R., 'Preselection of sex: the social consequences of choice', *The Sciences*, **20** (4) (April 1980) pp. 6–9 and 28.

Steinbacher, R., 'Futuristic implications of sex preselection', in Holmes, H. B., Hoskins, B. B., and Gross, M. (eds), *The Custom-Made Child? Women-Centered Perspectives* (Clifton, NJ: The Humana Press 1981), pp. 187–91.

Steinbacher, R., 'Sex preselection: from here to fraternity', in Gould, C. (ed.), *Beyond Domination: New Perspectives on Women and Philosophy* (Totowa, NJ: Rowman and Allenheld), pp. 274–82.

Tedeschi, J., and Reiss, M., 'Identities, the phenomenal self, and laboratory research', in Tedeschi, J. (ed.), *Impression Management Theory and Social Psychology Research* (New York: Academic Press 1981), pp. 3–22.

Uddenberg, N., Almgren, P. E., and Nilsson, A., 'Preference for sex of child among pregnant women', *Journal of Biosocial Science*, **3** (1971), pp. 267–80.

Westoff, C. F., and Rindfuss, R. R., 'Sex preselection in the United States', *Science*, **184** (1974), pp. 633–6.

Williamson, N. E., *Sons or Daughters: a cross-cultural survey of parental preferences* (Beverly Hills, CA: Sage Publications 1976).

Zimmerman, J., 'Technology and the future of women: haven't we met somewhere before?', *Women's Studies International Quarterly*, **4** (3) (1981), pp. 355–67.

5 What's 'new' about the 'new' reproductive technologies?

Renate Duelli Klein

'In one way – not much; in another – everything.' This might be an answer to the question 'What's "new" about the "new" reproductive technologies?' In the following pages I shall, on the one hand, point to some of the similar ideologies underlying the practice of both the 'old' and the 'new' reproductive technologies and, on the other, discuss in what ways, in my view, the *new* reproductive technologies are different and why I believe that they have the potential to significantly worsen the global position of women as a group.[1*]

First, some definitions. I define 'reproductive technologies' as the full range of biomedical/technical interferences during the process of procreation whether aimed at producing a child or preventing/terminating pregnancy. 'Old' technologies include mechanical contraception (e.g. the IUD, cap, diaphragm, sponge, condom and spermicide) and the various forms of hormonal contraception (e.g. the Pill, the injectable Depo Provera, the hormonal implant). 'Old' technologies also include female and male sterilization, abortion, and mechanical interferences at birth such as episiotomies (an incision to enlarge the vaginal opening) and Caesarian sections. 'New' reproductive technologies encompass pre-conception sex selection and post-conception sex determination techniques, artificial insemination, and the full gamut of 'test-tube' techniques: *in vitro* fertilization (e.g. the fertilization of an egg cell with sperm in a glass dish in the lab), embryo replacement, transfer and 'flushing', embryo freezing, and –

* Superior figures refer to the Notes section following this chapter.

yet to come – cloning and the artificial placenta: the 'glass womb'. They also comprise the increasing number of antenatal tests during 'normal' pregnancy such as amniocentesis, the alpha-foeto protein test, foetal monitoring by foetoscopy and sonogram/ultrasound, and at birth (e.g. epidural anaesthesia which 'knocks out' a birthing woman from the waist down).[2]

Whether 'old' or 'new', these procedures have in common that they represent an artificial invasion of the human body – predominantly the female body. Increasingly, more and more control is taken away from an individual's body and concentrated in the hands of 'experts' – the rapidly – and internationally – growing brigade of 'technodocs': doctors, scientists and pharmaceutical representatives (most of them male, white, and of Euro-American origin) who fiercely compete with one another on this 'new frontier' of scientific discovery and monetary profits.

Such developments, however, do not take place in a vacuum. They reflect the interests, needs and wishes of the powers that be. Consequently, assessment of the 'old' as well as the 'new' reproductive technologies must recognize them as powerful socio-economic and political instruments of control. Feminist research has well documented that over thousands of years the control of women's bodies, and in particular of our reproductive biology, has been a crucial factor in the oppression of women (as a social group and as individuals) by men.[3] Patriarchy past and present attempts to mould women in and to its image and thus usurp control over women's lives: in some countries women are tortured by genital mutilation, in others they are deformed by cosmetic surgery or restrictive clothing in the name of 'beauty'. (In yet others they are unwanted and thus eliminated before or at birth; see Madhu Kishwar's article in this volume.)

An analysis of reproductive technologies must expose the role they play in the multi-faceted exploitation and domination of women. This holds true for the 'old' as well as the 'new' ones. But the 'new' technologies, in my view, reinforce the degradation and oppression of women to an unprecedentedly horrifying degree. They reduce women to living laboratories: to 'test-tube women'.

Before the advent of the latest technological 'successes' it was women's *whole* bodies that could be forced into – or out of – having children (and this is without reference to the way in which our minds have been coerced into accepting this fate and being happy with it!).

For instance, in the West, motherhood – still regarded as women's 'true' and noblest vocation – is in reality given neither status and esteem nor *practical* support. It is one of the lowliest and least rewarded jobs, and our child-hating society turns mothering into a constant struggle with unsuitable, badly equipped buildings (e.g. shops, houses, public places), unfavourable work and training conditions, discriminatory educational opportunities, inadequate health care, and of course a host of related attitudes to mothers as 'unreliable' workers because of their responsibility to take care of their children's needs.

The new aspect of the new reproductive technologies is that now it is *parts* of women which are used – and abused – to control the reproduction of the human species. The technodocs have embarked on dissecting and marketing parts of women's bodies: eggs, wombs and embryos. Women are being dismembered – split into separate reproductive parts which can be reassembled, perhaps in a different order, perhaps using parts from different women. Woman has become – as Gena Corea aptly calls it – *The Mother Machine* (1985): an incubator; a vessel; a reproductive body. And 'man' is closer to being the procreator of the species – playing God – than ever.

Under the spell of the 'technological fix' – which has a solution for every problem – more and more techniques are being perfected to produce 'better' babies: sperm banks ensure the genetic perpetuation of the 'best' man ('best', one must ask, according to which values and for whom?); the *in vitro* fertilized embryo will soon be screened for genetic defects and often the 'right' sex (and what are the consequences if it is the 'wrong' sex?); then the 'best' suited 'maternal environment' (which is the language the technodocs use to describe a woman's womb) is chosen; the 'embryo carrier' – a technical term for a pregnant woman – can even be 'fixed up' with more than one embryo – no matter that she might have quadruplets to look after for the next fifteen years![4]

During pregnancy the 'right' of the foetus to become a 'normal' baby is protected against hazards from its mother. The pregnant woman is urged to undergo tests such as amniocentesis and ultrasound, the side-effects of which are far from being fully assessed and recognized. In the USA, the stage has already been reached that should a woman refuse the suggested tests, and a disabled baby be born, the new baby could *sue* the mother for negligence![5]

As with the 'old' technologies the rule with the 'new' ones is that the less women interfere with the medical experts, the better. The technologies are removed from women, further mystified by the use of technical jargon. There is an absence of explanation, counselling, and a lack of discussion about the unknown dangers of the technologies and alternatives. There is no discussion about the social construction of motherhood and the question of real 'choice' a woman has in a society that continues to equate 'real' woman with mother and wife (see Robyn Rowland's article in this volume). A woman's future and her reproductive fate is all in the experts' hands – and how could we be so unreasonable as to doubt that it wasn't all for women's 'own good'? The pain, however, is the woman's problem, whether physical, for instance in laparoscopies (the removal of eggs from the ovaries which ironically is called 'egg recovery'), or psychological, if again and again hopes for a child are dashed, for the *in vitro* fertilization success rate is only about 20 per cent of achieved egg fertilizations and about 13–15 per cent of actual births.[6] Any feeling of failure, sadness, or guilt which might occur after an abortion of an 'abnormal' foetus discovered by means of amniocentesis (a painful operation when performed between the sixteenth to twentieth week of pregnancy) – these are women's problems too.

The new technological experts 'help' women as patients to 'master' and cure our bodily deficiencies. Reproduction in all its stages has become fully institutionalized as a medical phenomenon. Often under the guise of the 'excitement' of the scientific discovery, the technodocs are tampering with the reproduction of the human species. They are about to 'conquer' another part of life that they do not have access to 'naturally', to consolidate their power over women in yet another area. The questions that feminists must ask loudly and everywhere are: Who makes the rules? Whose needs and interests are being catered for? Who profits from this control? Who benefits? And who pays the price?

Women's desires and needs, our experiences of our own bodies, are discredited and declared neurotic and hysterical or simply part of the 'disease' of being female. For years some of us have coped with heavy side-effects as we swallowed the pill, but were told that this was the price to pay for being sexually 'liberated'. So we continued loathing our own biology. (That it was sexual liberation on men's terms and *for* men took some time to sink in . . . .) Our well-being does not seem to matter much – except when our desires happen to coincide with those of the group in power. In other words, the infertile woman in the West is pitied and admitted to test-tube baby programmes (that is if she is heterosexual, preferably married or in a stable relationship, in a secure financial position and preferably white and able-bodied). After all, we are told, a 'real' woman has the 'right' to fulfil her 'biological urge' . . . never mind that her infertility is very likely to be caused by IUDs and other harmful contraceptives (Pfeffer and Woollett 1983; Corea 1985). Infertile women in the southern hemisphere (or ethnic minorities, lesbians and other 'outcasts' in the West) do not get the same compassionate response: there are no infertility clinics in Asia and Africa and it is tacitly assumed that the fewer wombs that produce babies, the better. . . . The focus in so-called 'Third World' countries (and among unwanted ethnic minorities in the western world) is on population control. Thousands of Third World women in their home countries and abroad are used as guinea pigs for research on 'quick and easy' contraceptives: injectable hormones (such as Depo Provera and Net-En) that last three months, hormonal implants (e.g. Norplant, the two-phase artificial hormone Levonorgestrol inserted in a tube in women's arms) that render us infertile for up to five years allow women *no* control at all, and if the treatment leads to bleeding, nausea, haemorrhaging and even sterility, then the fate of 'those' women does not seem to matter (Balasubrahmanyan 1984; Bunkle 1984). And hysterectomies are performed by the thousands and under abysmal hygienic circumstances irrespective of countless infections and deaths. In the USA, 800,000 hysterectomies per year are performed and the majority of them are on women of colour: eugenics under a new guise (Cook and Dworkin 1981).

At the same time elsewhere in the world (for example in Romania in 1984), it is impossible to get any contraceptives. Because the government wants more children, women are coerced into bearing children: childless couples have to pay extra taxes, divorce is made very difficult and abortion, which has been illegal since 1966 for women under 42 and with less than four children, is now punished with up to ten years in goal, despite terrible economic conditions.[7]

Thus some women are forced to have children – and others are forced to remain childless. Legal and respected is whatever the group in power declares to be 'right' for a specific group of people at a specific time. (And the rules can change overnight!) There is nothing new about that. When women refuse to obey, when we take the control in our own hands – as for example with menstrual extraction to forego the problem of a pregnancy,[8] or women-controlled self-insemination, or feminist pregnancy counselling and radical midwifery – such action is often called 'dangerous', 'immoral', 'irresponsible'. (The moralistic condemnation of surrogacy expressed by the public must be critically assessed in this light too. Surrogacy, as it is presently exercised in the USA by commercial agencies, *does* exploit women badly (Ince 1984). However, it could *theoretically* be in women's control as no high technology is needed.) And while much research money goes into further research on reproductive technologies, little effort is made to improve the health of women and children and the education of girls (especially in Third World countries). Infant mortality rises world-wide (Morgan 1984). Women are the world's poor, sick, illiterate, malnourished, starving and old – more vulnerable than ever to the so-called 'benefits' from the new technologies (Scott 1984). In addition to selling our bodies for sex the new reproductive technologies enable us to lease our wombs for money. Perhaps soon too we can sell our eggs: countless eggs are needed for experiments. And while in other areas *old* women are devalued, perhaps in this case even the ovaries of older women will do! As for the continuing research on the development of the artificial placenta . . . could the removed (800,000) wombs of 'live' women be useful study material?

The new technologies thrive. And women often collude with the technodocs: sometimes because of economic necessity; sometimes because of the need to survive – emotionally and physically. Sterilization at least ensures that a mother doesn't have to become a criminal to feed more mouths. An amniocentesis in a country where a girl-child is a curse enables a woman to have yet another abortion and will at least save her from more degradation from her family.[9] But sometimes women also collude because we have been brainwashed. The information and education we get is one-sided and male-centred and the hidden conviction creeps into our own minds that men and their technology must be better than our own body and our own experiences with it. Women are indeed in a lifelong process 'broken by men' (Janice Raymond's words, 1986) to accept patriarchy's norms as *the* norms (at best we can become 'equal' on *their* terms). Hence the time might come when women opt for having babies *outside* our wombs if we are assured that this is much safer and far more controllable than a growing embryo in our imperfect body. Disabled people who dare to be alive could be more stigmatized than ever.

Removing childbearing functions from women might lead the patriarchy into new heydays of power over women. I think the prospects for our future are gloomy. The question of the 'old' and the 'new' reproductive technologies is *not* an individual issue. I believe that it is at the core of women's lack of freedom and real choices and thus has a bearing on the status of all women – young and old, interested and uninterested in having children. It is violence against women in a new and frightening sense. As women are dismembered for science's sake in labs, and embryos are transferred, replaced, divided, frozen, flushed out from a temporary surrogate mother's womb and operated upon, in 'real' life violence against women increases daily. Worldwide, pornography flourishes. Profoundly disturbing horror scenes of rape, mutilation, murder and degradation of women appear in sex movies and on the video screens of millions of 'ordinary' people at home. They reveal the deep-rooted woman-hating nature of our societies. Hitler and his national-socialist breeding programmes are of our very recent past. The 'opportunities' to use the reproductive technologies in an attempt to 'purify' a race are limitless. 'Brave new world' is here and it's neither 'brave' nor really new. It's more of the same for women – but it's much more sophisticated and insidious. And it's far more dangerous: the new reproductive technologies could become 'the final solution to the woman question' (to use Robyn Rowland's term, 1984) in a not-so-science-fiction world. When the 'glass womb' is perfected, women as a group might be obsolete as childbearers.

However, having babies and raising children is not the only work women do. In fact, women perform two-thirds of the world's dirtiest labour for minimal pay.[10] As women's work has historically been the work that men don't want to do, it is unlikely that the unemployed men of the future will compete with women for the really demeaning jobs. Perhaps the men will switch to a new identity around 'life at home', and computer programmes with information on creative child-rearing will abound.[11] Men could thus become the 'perfect fathers' of their artificially conceived (perhaps cloned from one of their body cells?), artificially carried, and hence artificially delivered child.

And the women? I think in the year 2000 we could well be even poorer, in much worse jobs, and with even less freedom and fewer rights and resources than today. Among the things the next 'wave' of the women's movement might have to fight for, could be a woman's right to bear our own natural children: we could have lost control over the last part of the reproductive process: to decide if, when, and how to conceive, carry and give birth to children.

The prospect of being even further colonized by patriarchy is deeply alarming. But perhaps if women *know* about the dehumanizing and dangerous aspects of the new reproductive technologies we will say 'no' to the expert who tries to coerce us, inferring that the technologies are better than our own bodies. In order to distribute the information and devise directions for change we need to organize. We have little time as the international technology craze continues. We *must* fight back.

Notes

1 I am most grateful to Rita Arditti and Shelley Minden with whom I edited *Test-Tube Women. What Future for Motherhood* (1984), and I thank all its contributors, in particular Barbara Katz Rothman, Gena Corea, Rebecca Albury, Jane Murphy, Susan Ince, Scarlet Pollock, Vimal Balasubrahmanyan, Phillida Bunkle, Marsha Saxton, Ruth Hubbard, Robyn Rowland, Janice Raymond and Jalna Hanmer for their insightful, inspirational and courageous work. In addition, my warm thanks to Dale Spender for many hours of fascinating discussion on the subject of the new reproductive technologies and for reading this paper, and to Catherine Itzin and Christine Zmroczek for constructive comments.

2 Artificial insemination, usually listed among the 'new' reproductive technologies, strictly speaking deserves a category of its own as 'low' technology (the various forms of *in vitro* fertilization would then be 'high' technology). Especially in the practice of self-insemination where a woman herself inserts the sperm (from an unknown donor or a friend) with a syringe into her vagina, no further technological interference takes place (see Duelli Klein 1984). In fact, the woman is in control of the technology. This is different in the case where official sperm banks act as intermediaries and screen both the sperm donor and the female customer, but even so, the actual act of depositing the sperm remains equally 'low tech'.

3 For the best overview see Ehrenreich and English (1978).

4 As of January 1985 three 'sets of Test Tube Squads' (Timmins 1985) have been born: two in England and one in Australia.

5 See Ruth Hubbard's article in *Test-Tube Women* (1984), p. 344.
6 Carl Wood in 1984 quotes 13 per cent for Australia; Davies David in 1985 10–15 per cent for Britain. From Rowland (1985).
7 BBC 4, radio feature, London, 23 March 1984: see also Morgan (ed.) 1984 in the chapter on Romania, pp. 576–80.
8 The self-help technique of extracting the menstrual blood (and thus, if necessary, perform an early abortion) with a simple suction device called Del-em was invented by Lorraine Rothman of the Feminist Women's Health Center in Los Angeles (Gage 1979). The device was soon brand-marked as highly dangerous by the medical establishment. It is regrettable that no money seems to be invested into improving (if indeed necessary) the safety of the Del-em. Is it because it would give women control over their fertility?
9 The country in question is India. See Viola Roggenkamp's interview with an Indian woman (1984).
10 These are the by now well-known statistics published by the United Nations: 'While women represent over half of the world adult population and one-third of the official labour force, women perform for nearly two-thirds of all working hours and receive only one-tenth of the world income. Women also own less than one per cent of world property' (1980).
11 Dale Spender is currently doing research on 'Post-industrial Man' in which she is exploring the effects of the technological revolution on the socio-economic relationship between women and men.

Bibliography

Arditti, Rita, Duelli Klein, Renate, and Minden, Shelley, *Test-Tube Women. What Future for Motherhood?* (London and Boston: Pandora Press 1984).

Balasubrahmanyan, Vimal, 'Women as targets in India's family planning policy', in Arditti *et al.*, *Test-Tube Women* (1984), pp. 153–64.

Bunkle, Phillida, 'Calling the shots: the international politics of Depo Provera', in Arditti *et al.*, *Test-Tube Women* (1984), pp. 165–87.

Cook, Cynthia and Dworkin, Susan, 'Tough talk about unnecessary surgery', *Ms.* (October 1981), pp. 43–4.

Corea, Gena, *The Mother Machine* (New York: Harper and Row 1985).

Duelli Klein, Renate, 'Doing it Ourselves: Self-Insemination', in Arditti *et al.*, *Test-Tube Women* (1984), pp. 382–90.

Ehrenreich, Barbara, and English, Deirdre, *For Her Own Good* (Garden City, New York: Anchor Press 1978).

Gage, Suzann, *When Birth Control Fails ... How to Abort Ourselves Safely* (Hollywood, California: Speculum Press 1979).

Ince, Susan, 'Inside the surrogate industry', in Arditti *et al.*, *Test-Tube Women* (1984), pp. 99–116.

Morgan, Robin (ed.), *Sisterhood is Global* (Garden City, New York: Anchor Press/Doubleday 1984).

Pfeffer, Naomi, and Woollett, Anne, *The Experience of Infertility* (London: Virago 1983).

Raymond, Janice, *Female Friendship. A Philosophy* (Boston: Beacon Press, forthcoming 1986).

Rowland, Robyn, 'Reproductive Technologies: the final solution to the woman question?', in Arditti *et al.*, *Test-Tube Women* (1984), pp. 356–70.

Rowland, Robyn, 'A Child at ANY Price? An overview of issues in the use of the new reproductive technologies and the threat to women', *Women's Studies International Forum*, **8** (5) in press (1985).

Scott, Hilda, *Working Your Way to the Bottom. The Feminization of Poverty* (London and Boston: Pandora Press 1984).

Timmings, Nicholas, 'Third test-tube quads born', *The Times* (29 January 1985).

United Nations, 'Program of Action for 2nd Half of the U.N. Decade for Women. Equality, Development and Peace', Item 9 of the Provisional Agenda 80–12383, World Conference of the United Nations Decade for Women, Copenhagen, Denmark (1980).

6 Motherhood, patriarchal power, alienation and the issue of 'choice' in sex preselection

Robyn Rowland

This paper explores the relationship between women's demand for choice in reproduction and sexuality; our attitudes towards motherhood; male control of conception and reproduction; and sex preselection technology. It tentatively raises the possibility that 'choice' and 'freedom' as a continuing ideological base in the area of reproductive technology may eventually entrap women further and limit their choice to say 'no' to increased male control of the reproductive process. It makes the distinct point that feminists *must* educate themselves in this field and *must* re-evaluate the issues of reproductive freedom and the 'right to choose' in terms of the long-term consequences of uncontrolled medical 'advances'.

The motivation for this presentation of such a complex interaction of ideas comes from three sources of concern to me at present. First, I have been researching and talking with infertile couples who seek artificial insemination. This has meant contact for over two years with the medical team running the foremost *in vitro* fertilization (IVF) programme in operation, led by Carl Wood. This team has moved within the reproductive area at rapid speed, leaving debate by social groups and ethics committees lagging. It has the highest rate of pregnancies; conducts IVF with donor ova and donor sperm; has frozen embryos (two pregnancies to date); and is about to try a new technique of 'flushing' an embryo from a donor woman. The work is conducted within a social milieu generally ignorant of both the medical and social consequences of these techniques. When the state government placed a brief moratorium on the use of donor eggs, and when they attempted to suspend the frozen embryo scheme, women patients took the government to the Equal Opportunity Board, demanding their right of access to this technology. Doctors claim that their primary reason for continuing this research is that 'women want it'.

Second, my problems with existing technologies made me extend my vision to consider the technologies foreshadowed but not yet in use: sex preselection, cloning and ectogenesis (use of artificial womb/placenta) (see Rowland 1984). It is clear that the legal, social, medical and policy debates within the IVF area should have been conducted *before* the techniques were offered to infertile women. Society finds it impossible to withdraw access to a technology once it is available, regardless of its negative consequences. We therefore need to consider policy *now* for foreshadowed technology.

Third, there is a renewed interest in motherhood within a previously disenchanted women's movement. Many lesbian and single women are adopting children, or more frequently, using artificial insemination to conceive. To many feminists the new technology offers a positive solution to both infertility in women and to childbearing without heterosexual relations.

But women are again assuming a benign medicine. The medical profession in fact fails to differentiate between research to aid infertility and research to change and control conception and the genetic balance. It is again using women's bodies for experimentation and using their 'need' (social or otherwise) to have babies. Women, motivated by an intense life crisis over infertility, are manipulated by this situation into full and total support of any technique which will produce those desired children, without consideration of the implications of doing so for women as a social group.

I have argued elsewhere that if we continue in this framework, sex preselection, cloning and ectogenesis, combined with surrogate motherhood, will ensure that the fragility of women's power is worn to gossamer and finally fades. Much as we turn from consideration of a nuclear aftermath, we turn from seeing a future where children are neither borne nor born or where women are forced to bear only sons and to slaughter their foetal daughters. Chinese and Indian women are already trudging this path. The future of women as a group is at stake and we need to ensure that we have thoroughly considered all possibilities before endorsing technology which could mean the death of the female.

Pro-natalist ideology

Pro-natalist ideology, whether controlled or uncontrolled, is basic to most countries today. Having babies is necessary, as long as women do it where, when and how often social mores or laws decree. Feminist ideology is also experiencing a return to pro-natalist values, though with the desire to change the institution of motherhood as designed by patriarchal ideology.

One of the first moves of the renewed women's movement of the 1960s was to reject the advice of 'experts' with respect to childcare. Spurred on by the belief that 'maternal instinct' is a social construct not a biological destiny, women discovered through 'rap' and CR groups that 'expert' advice did not fit with women's experience. Bowlby had scared a generation of women into thinking that if they left their child for even brief periods, trauma would result. Though it cost them a great deal in guilt, women rejected those advisers.

'Maternity is natural' also trapped women into the nuclear family, which came to be seen as a fortress of male dominance. Married women were chained through it to a dependent existence: they worked for no wage, and little job security, could be sexually exploited or abused with the sanction of the law, and had the status of a minor. Within this context there was no choice for women, and 'choice' was the focal point of the movement.

A variety of causes were seen to guide women into motherhood. They had children because they were socialized or conditioned to do so, and were convinced of the rewards of mothering; in order to gain a self-identity in a world which continually denied this to them; to prove their worth and attain the status of an 'adult'. For many, motherhood represented a power base from which to negotiate the terms of their existence and survival, and for many this is still the case.

Many women began to make a choice to remain childless and became partners in childfree relationships. In 1972, Shulamith Firestone wrote in the *Dialectic of Sex*: 'Pregnancy is barbaric ... the temporary deformation of the body of the individual for the sake of the species' (p. 88). Women, she said, should be freed from 'the tyranny of reproduction by every means possible' (p. 193).

Mary O'Brien in her analysis *The Politics of Reproduction* (1981) comments that traditional wisdom had said: 'Women are naturally trapped in the childbearing function/women therefore cannot participate in social life on equal terms with men' (p. 20). In place of this, she says, feminists like De Beauvoir and Firestone claimed: 'Women are naturally trapped in the childbearing function/therefore the liberation of women depends on their being freed from this trap'

(p. 20). To Firestone, this freedom was only possible if women were liberated from maternity through use of a test-tube baby system.

In recent years, however, a further re-evaluation of the value of maternity has begun. Many feminists are seeking now to recreate the experience of motherhood and family in a non-exploitative way. Works such as those by Elisabeth Badinter (1981) and Ann Dally (1982) have helped to clarify the *mythology* of motherhood as opposed to the *experience* women have of motherhood. Badinter analyses the development of 'maternal instinct' as a construct, showing that 'no *universal and absolute* conduct on the part of the mother has emerged' (p. 327).

In *Of Woman Born. Motherhood as Experience and Institution* (1977) Adrienne Rich explores the institution of motherhood as it has been controlled by men and patriarchal society to the point where it has become a distorted experience for women. It is this institutionalization of motherhood which is the problem, not the experience itself. Women have been divorced from their bodies by the mythologizing of them on the one hand, and the downgrading of them on the other. Mindful always of the danger of the biological determinism argument, she moves beyond it to point out that we are in fact our bodies as well as mind, spirit and intellect, but how we define that relationship should be in the control of women, not of men.

Mary O'Brien in *The Politics of Reproduction* (1981) argues that feminists have been too ready to cut reproduction out of their lives because of its history of entrapment, and we should in fact be using it as a starting point of a new political theory: to redefine an understanding of gender relations *beginning* at reproduction. O'Brien writes: 'I argue that it is from an adequate understanding of the process of reproduction, nature's traditional and bitter trap for the suppression of women, that women can begin to understand their possibilities and their freedom' (p. 9). She claims that men have their rituals and ritualistic meetings which reinforce them as 'male' but women lack this particular structure. To celebrate being 'female', O'Brien claims we need some rituals, and the birth experience is a primary one which in the past was shared with other women. But this has been broken by the intervention of medicine in birth.

O'Brien goes on to discuss what she calls 'reproductive consciousness'. In her terms, the first significant historical change was the discovery of physiological paternity which transformed male reproductive consciousness: men discovered that they were, in fact, the seed. The second and more recent change in reproductive consciousness was triggered by technology in the form of contraception, which gave women the freedom to choose or reject parenthood.

The fact that men provide the seed in reproduction however, also ensures their alienation from 'genetic continuity', i.e., 'unlike the other role – the necessity to produce – the reproductive role resists male participation and control' (p. 33). Because women bear the child and 'labour' at birth, they have the certainty of their essential participation in the genetic continuity. The way in which men have always annulled their alienation from reproduction is described by O'Brien as the 'appropriation of the child' (p. 36). Thus by law or by force, men appropriate and control women and children. This is intended to eliminate their 'uncertainty' in the reproductive process.

O'Brien sees this alienation experience reflected in obstetrics, to which men have brought 'the sense of their own alienated parental experience of reproduction, and have translated this into the forms and languages of an "objective science"' (p. 46). The power men have claimed to make themselves 'the universal' and women 'the other' has enabled them to keep women isolated from each other, to break their culture, and to exclude them from power: 'all of these have obscured the cultural consciousness of femininity and the universality of maternal consciousness' (p. 50). The female reproductive consciousness is thus seen as universal and common to all women, mothers or not, as it represents an understanding of our place in the continuity of life, which is explored through our physiology (but not that alone), and is reinforced by, for example, menstruation, menopause and pregnancy.

Chodorow, in her book *The Reproduction of Mothering* (1978), traces the way mothering is passed on from mother to daughter. She writes that women by and large want to mother, and get gratification from their mothering; and finally, that, with all the conflicts and contradictions, women have succeeded at mothering (p. 7). And in her article on 'Maternal thinking', Ruddick analyses the qualities of thinking and caring which enforced mothering has in fact developed in women. Thus, though the practices of mothering are oppressive, at its best, the qualities of mothering or maternal thinking embody the kind of caring we would wish men to express to others. They stand in opposition to the destructive, violent and self-aggrandizing characteristics of men.

Invitation to men

There is, within the reappraisal of motherhood, an invitation to men to participate more fully in parenting. Ruddick insists that the only way of introducing maternal values into the political domain is to assimilate men into the private domain of childcare. This would break down the separation of the two spheres, take the pressure off women to live vicariously through their children; and give men an investment in making the public domain more committed to reforming childcare procedures. However, she also warns: 'But in our eagerness, we mustn't forget that so long as a mother is not effective publicly and self-respecting privately, male presence can be harmful as well as beneficial' (1980: p. 361).

Badinter also concludes that the difference between giving birth and having the sole responsibility for rearing the child have been conveniently confused by patriarchy and that this is the key to women's oppression. She places faith in what she sees as the emergence of 'father love' in 'the history of feelings' (p. 322). Women are demanding that men share in the love for a child and in her/his development. 'Henceforth', she says, 'women will "force" men to be good fathers, to share equitably the pleasures and burdens, the anxieties and sufferings of mothering' (p. 325). Though these conclusions have a utopian aura, they are shared by many women who have managed to involve the father of their child more fully in parenting, and by those who still struggle to do so. However, one statement within her vision has worrying overtones:

> Under the pressure exerted by women, the new father mothers equally and in the traditional mother's image. *He creeps in like another mother, between the mother and the child*, who experiences almost indiscriminately as intimate a contact with the father as the mother. (p. 324; my stress.)

O'Brien also sees a role for men in the solution to these conflicts. She writes:

> Finally, the integration of women on equal terms into the productive process is a necessary but not significant condition of liberation. Liberation also depends on the reintegration of men on equal terms into the reproductive process. (p. 210.)

It should be stressed, however, that this desire to include men more fully takes place in a society in which the structures and power dynamics of the family have changed little if at all.

Furthermore, the reproductive processes of which these women write involve an assumed 'natural' conception through sexual intercourse. The rapidity with which reproductive technology and engineering is taking place is changing the origin of conception for many individuals. I have outlined elsewhere the development of cloning and ectogenesis (artificial womb/placenta). These technologies open the way for greater male control over both conception and reproduction. Edward Grossman (1971) for example, has staunchly supported development of the artificial womb, listing the following advantages: foetal medicine would be improved(!); the child could be immunized while still inside the 'womb'; the environment would be *safer* than a woman's womb; geneticists could programme-in some superior trait; sex preselection would be simple; women would be 'spared the discomfort' of childbirth; women could be permanently sterilized; and men would be able to prove for the first time who is the father of the child.

Issues of a benign medicine

If these technologies were in the hands of women whose bodies they most intimately affect, we may be able to utilize them to free women and give them new choices. But past experience teaches us that the control of women's bodies is a continual battleground of the sexes. We are constantly being used as 'living laboratories' and suffer the consequences. Mary Daly in *Gyn/ecology* (1978) and Ehrenreich and English (1976) in *For Her Own Good* have clearly outlined this history, showing the appropriation of medicine by men, the elimination of women healers, and the resulting exploitation of women through their bodies.

The Pill was hailed once as the true liberator of women, yet its resulting 'freedom' is now viewed with suspicion and scepticism by feminists. It ensured that most women users had control over their fertility; but also that they were then 'at fault' if they became pregnant. It allowed men to become less responsible and women to become targets for sexual use more readily. In addition, it led to higher rates of cancer and thrombosis, and continues to be a drug which is taken on the basis of little and poor research into its side-effects. Depo Provera, the most 'efficient' contraception, has placed many women at risk. The Dalkon Shield, a contraceptive inter-uterine device (IUD), has in fact caused deaths of women through infection and septic abortion, and represents again the use of women's bodies by a medicine little concerned for the well-being of its victims. Can we assume that sex preselection will be an equivalent 'advance' in women's reproduction freedom?

Issues in sex preselection: the effects

That societies in general are male-preferring has been clearly demonstrated in a number of studies (e.g. Fidell, Hoffman and Keith-Spiegal 1979; Williamson 1976; Horn 1984). Even within educated groups the majority of people would choose male offspring as first-borns. Few are female *preferring*, but are disinterested rather than selective (Steinbacher 1981). In addition, Hartley and Pietraczk found in a group of 2138 Americans a 'widespread acceptance of ongoing biomedical research to perfect preselection methods' and a strong indication of intent to use such methods were they to become available.

The variety of techniques available now has been clearly outlined by this panel. They range from those necessitating abortion to those intended to preselect during conception (or to use Janice Raymond's term, to previctimize women).

The advantages and disadvantages of its availability have also been clearly outlined. Table 1 is based on Fletcher's (1983) table with some additions.

On the positive side it is assumed that because most societies are male-preferring, those born girls will feel specially wanted. People will easily limit family size instead of trying for a boy or girl after two or three of the one sex. Families will also be happier because there will be no disappointment at the birth of a 'wrong' sex child. The over-populated countries which are more strongly male-preferring will be able to control their population more easily through making choice available. (Is this a naïve assumption of availability of this technology in poorer nations?)

Some have suggested that woman's status will rise. Because of her scarcity woman will be 'highly-valued'. However, she will be valued for sexual and breeding purposes rather than for her intrinsic worth as

Table 1 Possible positive and negative consequences of sex preselection

	Positive		*Negative*
1	Avoidance of sex-linked disease	1	Mainly the rich will benefit
2	Girls will feel especially wanted	2	Wherever a strong boy preference, girls will be present in fewer numbers
3	Balance two-child family	3	Concentration of first- and second-born characteristics in boys or girls
4	Enhance happiness in families	4	Imbalance of sex ratio and social dislocation
5	Reduce population in less-developed nations	5	Precedent for genetic engineering, eugenics
6	Enhance family planning	6	Increase conflict between sexes
7	Increase human control over genetics	7	Possibility of abuse by totalitarian state
8	Increase status of women	8	Impact of expectations on the child

a person. 'When women are scarce and men readily available', write Guttenberg and Secord (1983), 'a protective morality develops that favours monogamy for women, limits their interactions with men, and shapes female roles in traditional domestic directions' (p. 231).

On the negative side, only the rich will have access to the technology. I would add that, as with IVF, single, lesbian, minority and poor women will have difficulty affording the technology. The concentration of boys as firstborns will also ensure that sexual stereotypes are firmly embedded in biology: firstborns tend to be more independent, achieving, active, dominant and successful (see Steinbacher and Holmes in this volume).

The imbalance of the sex ratio has been hypothesized as leading to a rise in 'male' values: aggression, sexual pressure on women, alcoholism and violence. As Campbell wrote: 'more of everything, in short, that men do, make, suffer, inflict and consume' (1976: p. 88).

Postgate (1973) has suggested that women's right to work will need to be curtailed and polyandry would develop. Some societies 'might treat their women as queen ants, others as rewards for the most outstanding (or most determined) males' (p. 16). In fact, it is likely that 'choice' of sexual partner will not be allowed as men demand and take sexual satisfaction and breeding rights from the diminishing numbers of women. I would suggest that female suicide rates would escalate.

Women are the most exploited, manipulated, oppressed and brutalized group in the world, yet we have the numbers. What would our status be as a vastly outnumbered group? And how many women would be prepared to accept a world where their value as breeders or sexual objects only would be recognized?

The issue of eugenics is also primary. Sex preselection technology is so closely related to genetic research, that manipulation of the genetic pool could follow. 'Breeding in' or out certain characteristics may creep in. In Australia, genetic manipulation of sheep has advanced to the point where they can be bred to twice their size with an increased wool yield (Roberts 1984). Animal research is less scrutinized than human work, yet it forms the basis of reproductive work with humans.

The possibility of the use of these techniques by a state imposing its will on women has already been realized in China (Mosher 1984). Mosher estimates that the limit of one child per family has resulted in enforced abortion to the rate of 10 million abortions annually through the 1970s. These are not only abortions in the first twelve weeks, but by injection to kill the foetus followed by Caesarian at seven or eight months. The most frequent contraceptive method (enforced) is female sterilization, as men equate vasectomy with castration. As China is a male-preferring and male-dominant society, sex preselection would have obvious consequences for the female foetus.

And finally, in all these discussions the experience of the child who grows to adulthood as the result of preselected sex is rarely discussed. They would carry the burden of their parents' desires and expectations which were attached to a particular sex. As with children born of AID and IVF programmes, a great deal of stress will be placed upon them to 'perform' in order not to disappoint their parents and make them wish they had 'chosen otherwise'.

Issues in sex preselection: choice, freedom and control

One of the tenets of the women's movement has been the issue of choice with respect to sexuality and reproduction. We demanded the right to *choose* whether to have children or not: and got contraception and abortion rights for many. This was double-edged as indicated earlier, but still gave some women increased choice. We then demanded the right to *have* children. Pfeffer and Woollett (1983) have stressed that the right to have children for infertile women is as imperative a right as that of being childfree. And medicine has provided ways – expensive and dangerous – for infertile women to do this.

Past choices *opened* opportunities for women *as a social group*. But what of a 'choice' which *closes* opportunities to women as a social group? Does the desire, the need, the wanting of choice have *no* boundaries? There must be a time at which the rights of one group impinge so strongly on those of the majority that social control is needed. Then the terminology of 'rights' becomes meaningless. Powledge (1983) would argue that the principal of freedom of choice must be second to that of 'fairness' and equal treatment.

It may be that the stress on choice gives the medical profession more not less control in the reproductive technology area. The 'right' to choose the sex of your child; the 'right' to use donor ova; the 'right' to have a surrogate mother and the 'right' of the medical profession to *service* these rights, have been used to ensure a lack of government and social intervention. And that *is* what we wanted with abortion and contraception and in sexuality. But is it what we want with reproductive technology that changes the sex ratio or clones human beings or changes genetic structure? Should people have the right to choose their child's genetic make-up, for example, or manipulate it to their desired prototype? What is 'the right to choose' in this context? Gordon (1979) has pointed out that 'we cannot always distinguish our personal need for the product from the "needs" defined for us by social policy' (p. 119).

Perhaps a useful distinction is that abortion gives women control over our bodies and our lives. Sex preselection gives men control over the sex of the next generation. We do not live in an ideological vacuum. We do live in a society in which men make the decisions. Within the dyadic and social power structures, the coercive power of man could be used to ensure the sex of *their* choice in offspring.

Powledge is one of the few feminists to tackle public policy on this question. She argues that reproductive freedom is subsidiary to the goal of equal treatment. If reproductive freedom invalidates 'fairness' it becomes secondary. She does not, however, advocate legal restrictions on reproductive freedom even if a technology will be used selectively against women, because of the risks that it will be generalized and place other reproductive freedoms, like abortion, at risk. Medicine, she claims, is also an 'inappropriate (and ineffective) locus of moral control' (p. 210). Some areas where control can be placed is on the research area itself, 'eliminating targeted research' by withdrawal of funding. And if advances in the field occur unexpectedly, as is often the case, controls would have to be imposed *ad hoc*, on the *application* of the research findings.

Policy decisions may have to be made in the reproductive area which will contradict current feminist ideology on reproductive freedom or expand it in a new direction. We have a responsibility, not just to women who want children and who may be infertile, but to the generations of people who will be the results of the use of new technology. To retain control over human experimentation, women may have to consider state intervention of some kind in the areas of research funding, research application and reproductive rights – with all its inherent dangers. Feminists may have to consider alignments with strange pillow-friends: right-wing women perhaps? We may have to call for an end to research which would have helped infertile women to conceive, in consideration of the danger to women as a social group of loss of control over 'natural' childbearing (e.g. the right *not* to choose the sex of your child).

Denise Riley (1981) has commented that 'relations between the State, population policies (whether pro or anti-natalist), feminism and the "right to choose" stand directly, at an interface between individual rights and government policy' (p. 185). This is an uncomfortable position for us but the dilemma must be debated and considered. The private versus public domain conflict arises here again.

When we extend our vision to include sex preselection, cloning and ectogenesis, we must question whether in supporting, pursuing or allowing reproductive technology to advance at its current pace, without real control and in the hands of male-dominated medicine and the drug companies, women are helping to create a situation where choice produces conflict, stress and the ultimate establishment of stereotypes in biology.

Hanmer and Allan (1980) have said that women act as agents of male individual and social power. We continue to collude to our own disadvantage. We need to challenge our own thinking and the current technology without eroding the hard-won gains we have made in reproductive choice. In the end, does the new technology mean a transfer of *power* to women as a social group? Or are they methods by which men gain their desired control over reproduction and conception itself, thus terminating their 'alienation' from the process, while increasing women's alienation? It is worthwhile to keep in mind Roberta Steinbacher's comments on the contraceptive pill: 'Who invented it, who manufactures it, who licensed it, who dispenses it? But who dies from it?' (1981: p. 89).

References

Arditti, Rita, Duelli Klein, Renate, and Minden, Shelley (eds), *Test-Tube Women. What future for motherhood?* (London and Boston: Pandora Press 1984).

Badinter, Elizabeth E., *The Myth of Motherhood. An historical view of the maternal instinct* (London: Souvenir Press 1981).

Campbell, Colin, 'The Manchild Pill', *Psychology Today*, August 1976, pp. 86–91.

Chodorow, Nancy, *The Reproduction of Mothering. Psychoanalysis and the sociology of gender* (Berkeley: University of California Press 1978).

Daly, Mary, *Gyn/ecology. The metaethics of radical feminism* (Boston: Beacon Press 1978).

Dally, Ann, *Inventing Motherhood. The consequences of an ideal* (London: Burnett Books 1982).

Ehrenreich, Barbara, and English, Deidre, *For Her Own Good. 150 years of the experts' advice to women* (New York: Anchor Books 1978).

Fidell, L., Hoffman, D., and Keith-Spiegel, P., 'Some social implications of sex-choice technology', *Psychology of Women Quarterly*, **4** (1) (1979) pp. 32–42.

Firestone, Shulamith, *The Dialectic of Sex* (London: Paladin 1972).

Fletcher, J. C., 'Ethics and public policy: should sex choice be discouraged?', in Bennett, N. (ed.), *Sex Selection of Children* (New York: Academic Press 1983).

Gordon, Linda, 'The struggle for reproductive freedom: three stages of feminism', in Z. Eisenstein (ed.), *Capitalist Patriarchy and the case for*

Socialist Feminism (New York: Monthly Review Press 1979).
Grossman, Edward, 'The Obsolescent Mother. A scenario', *The Atlantic*, **227** (1971), pp. 39–50.
Guttenberg, M., and Secord, P., *Too Many Women? The sex ratio question* (London: Sage 1983).
Hanmer, Jalna, and Allen, Pat, 'Reproductive engineering: The final solution?', *Feminist Issues*, **2** (1982), pp. 53–75.
Hartley, S. F., and Pietraczk, L., 'Preselecting the sex of offspring: technologies, attitudes and implications', *Social Biology*, **20** (1979), pp. 232–46.
Horn, P., 'Parents still prefer boys', *Psychology Today* (1984), pp. 19–30.
Mosher, Steve, 'The Truth about China', *The National Times* (Australia) (2–8 March 1984), pp. 25–9.
O'Brien, Mary, *The Politics of Reproduction* (London: Routledge & Kegan Paul 1984).
Pfeffer, Naomi, and Woollett, Ann, *The experience of infertility* (London: Virago 1983).
Postgate, John, 'Bat's chance in hell', *New Scientist*, 5 (1973), pp. 11–16.
Powledge, Tabitha, 'Towards a moral policy for sex choice', in Bennett, N. (ed.), *Sex Selection of Children* (1983).
Rich, Adrienne, *Of Woman Born. Motherhood as experience and institution* (London: Virago 1977).
Riley, Denise, 'Feminist thought and reproductive control: the State and "the right to choose"', in *Women in Society*, Cambridge Women's Studies Group (London: Virago 1981).
Roberts, Peter, 'Soon a super sheep', *Age*, Australia, Melbourne (5 March 1984).
Rowland, Robyn, 'Reproductive technologies: the Final solution to the women problem?', in Arditti, et al., *Test-Tube Women (1984).*
Ruddick, Sara, 'Maternal thinking', Feminist Studies, **6** (1980), pp. 342–67.
Steinbacher, Roberta, 'Futuristic implications of sex preselection', in Holmes, H., Hoskins, B., and Gross, M. (eds), *The Custom-made child? Women-centred perspectives* (New Jersey: Humana Press 1981).
Williamson, Nancy, *Sons or daughters. A cross-cultural survey of parental preferences* (London: Sage 1976).

7 Transforming consciousness: women and the new reproductive technologies

Jalna Hanmer

Could our certainty about the part played by women in the reproduction of children be shaken? Could the 'naturalness' on which this rests be challenged – even made as uncertain as our understanding, or consciousness, is of women's sexuality today? If this were to happen, what would be the implications for our understanding of ourselves as women?

These questions are concerned with consciousness. What impact is science and technology having on women's consciousness – through the new reproductive technologies – now and in the future? To explore these questions I look at how sexuality, childcare and biological reproduction began to be conceived, and acted upon, as separate rather than indivisible attributes and activities of women. While it is arbitrary to limit consideration of technological interventions to the past fifteen years, it was during this time that women collectively began to take up issues around sexuality, childcare and biological reproduction. One way of examining the implications of the new reproductive technologies for women is to relate the practical concerns of the present wave of the women's movement with recent technological innovations aimed at women's bodies – and to recall the various stages of the earlier struggles by women to overthrow dominant ideology through the development of revolutionary consciousness.

First I look at how women's consciousness altered around sexuality and recall the impact of scientific research into the sexual and reproductive biology of women. Then I look at the demand for control over our bodies, perhaps the most fundamental of all the demands of the women's liberation movement. On the one hand, women desired 'choice'. To have or not have children and to conceive and deliver children in self-determined ways. On the other hand, the state – through its medical services – encouraged some women to have children and discouraged others, while increasing technological interventions. Then I look at how the progressive takeover of the process of biological reproduction by men through science and medicine may affect the consciousness of both men and women. I then look at the theoretical questions women are asking and solutions they are offering about childcare and biological reproduction. A major aim is to relate the changes in women's consciousness around sexuality to what may happen to women's consciousness around reproduction. I conclude with why consciousness is our most important defence.

Identity and consciousness are key concerns of the present wave of feminism. 'What is a woman?' merges with 'Who am I?' In the early days of the women's liberation movement (WLM), the emphasis was on raising consciousness about the life experiences of women. The aim was to begin a process of seeing in a new way, of destroying old certainties by probing half-forgotten, unsettled experiences. More subtle than the Marxist project of overcoming false consciousness, the process involves a reinterpretation of everyday life. Bartky characterizes the process as realizing that what is happening is quite different from what *appears* to be happening; a process which is frequently followed by the inability to tell what really is happening at all (Bartky 1977). The youth resistance of the late 1960s sloganized, 'do not adjust your mind, reality is at fault'. The old certainties dissolve; inner divisions become conscious and women experience ourselves as 'victim and whose victimisation determines her being-in-the-world as resistance, wariness and suspicion' (Bartky 1977: p. 32).

Consciousness-raising led to a questioning of the 'natural' facts of sex and gender, thereby exposing inequalities between men and women in every aspect of life. In dominant ideology female sexuality, biological reproduction and childrearing are inextricably linked 'natural' activities in which women are dependent on men. The present wave of the women's movement began to question this conflation and its inherent biologism. The 'naturalness' of wifehood and motherhood was challenged through the development of feminist activity and analysis.

While there always have been methods of contraception and abortion (McLaren 1985), the assumption that sexuality and reproduction are indivisible received a serious blow with hormonal contraception;

that is, the Pill. The Pill helped to launch the 'swinging sixties' and aided the recognition that sexuality is separate from biological reproduction and childrearing, which remained securely linked through the concept of motherhood.

While some women came into the women's liberation movement as lesbians, and others were, and remain, heterosexual, many women began to question their sexuality at this time. The so-called sexual revolution diversified and legitimated heterosexual practices and experiences, changing understandings of what it is to be a sexual woman (Brunt 1982). Abandoning the missionary posture, discovering masturbation, a counter-cultural hippy wave of 'Do It', ended for many women in the exploration of their sexuality with other women. Consciousness-raising around their life experiences had exposed the oppressiveness of sexual politics.

Around the same time research into the physiology of female sexuality undermined widely held beliefs derived from the work of Freud (Masters and Johnson 1966). While not unknown to some individuals, they established experimentally that the clitoris is *the* site of female sexual pleasure. Stimulating women through a specially constructed machine established the 'scientific' nature of this knowledge. The unchallenged and unchallengeable dogma of Freud that 'mature' women move their erogenous zone from the clitoris to the vagina, thereby making lesbian sexuality 'immature', collapsed. As Jill Johnston wrote, women reacted 'As though the case for an insensitive vagina provided women with their first legal brief for the indictment of phallic imperialism' (1973: p. 169). The old certainties that women's sexual gratification depends solely upon men through heterosexual relations receded, leaving the social space necessary for rethinking, through experimentation, the nature of female sexuality.

What is 'natural' about it, we asked? Can a 'truer' female sexuality be experienced with other women? The exposure of the true site of female sexual enjoyment fed the belief that society is a social construct, as are the individuals who make it up. How *could* we have been taken in by Freud? The plasticity of people, the ability to socially mould personal gender and sexual characteristics came home to many women through experiencing for the first time female sexual enjoyment with women. Women left men for women, giving their emotional and sexual selves to their sisters.

The present wave of the women's liberation movement began as an analysis of so-called private life through consciousness-raising that often ended in lesbianism – that is, the belief that women are the proper objects of love and care for women. For many women the logical conclusion of the analytic and personal challenge to men (whatever their political stances), embodied in the slogan 'the personal is political', was to become more closely identified with women individually and as a social group, that is, to become women-identified-women. The rebonding of women with each other led to the study of the history of female friendships (Faderman 1981). But the belief began to grow that women are so moulded by the social dominance of men that we will never know how women in a true state of nature (whatever that is) experience their sexuality.

The history of how men appropriated women's sexuality so that it became a slavish attention to male sexual needs began to be studied (Coveney *et al.* 1984). The so-called purity campaigns of the latter half of the nineteenth century are being reassessed. Women's demands that men exercise self-control, that they be chaste, were a response to the impact of male sexuality on women and girls. Feminists made a resolute attack on the double standard; an accepted code of practice that enabled men to sow their wild oats but held women responsible for any deviation from virginity before marriage and monogamy thereafter. Dominant ideology was under fire and in the ensuing struggle Havelock Ellis became the major theoretician shifting understanding of the problem from male licentiousness to female frigidity.

This ideological shift was only possible because the material conditions of women changed. The deal, so to speak – the siting of the problem on women and not on men – was made possible by improved contraception. The agony of unchecked male sexuality and its consequences in childbirth for married women, always the most numerous group subject to heterosexuality, is recounted, for example, in the letters sent to the secretary of the Co-operative Society just before the First World War (Davies 1915). Rubber technology gave greater control over fertility to individual women who could obtain the diaphragm or who could encourage their men to use the sheath.

More effective birth control methods served to delegitimate both women's refusal of sex with men because of fear of pregnancy and their criticism of men's sexuality as in need of control. Much later hormonal contraception, and legal abortion, removed these same 'excuses' from unmarried women, creating the social space for the so-called sexual revolution of the 1960s. This is not to assume that all women had equal access to these methods, or that the decline in the birth rate was without fluctuations, or that sex refusal reasoning was effective in practice. Women still ended up with children and the long-term consequences of caring and childrearing. These improvements in contraception, however, invalidated sex refusal. Women no longer had any reason for 'not liking it'. Women who did not were declared frigid, a psychological condition deemed in need of treatment by the medical, psychological, psychiatric and social work professions and women began to be treated for what has become a medicalized condition.

The critique of sexuality that began with consciousness-raising in the late 1960s, however, challenged the 'naturalness' of the view that women 'ought' to like sexual relations with men and if they did not, they suffered from an abnormality called frigidity. The discovery of a time before Ellis, the purity movement and the sex reformers, when females were viewed as sexual, even possibly more highly sexed than men, further exposed the degree of social conditioning of a so-called natural biological urge.

Exposure of these cultural manipulations of the nature of female sexuality transforms the conscious understanding of women. On the one hand, increased consciousness is a way of developing a sense of self through re-evaluating experience which includes intellectually acquired knowledge. On the other hand, how can we be certain that the place we are now in is any more 'natural'? Or more truly expressive of our 'real' self? With each exposure of social deception women's consciousness of themselves as sexual beings controlling the expression of their own sexuality, is made more uncertain. This is the price to be paid for increased consciousness when women live in conditions of servitude, even slavery, always in second place socially and, more often than not, in their personal relationships in marriage and family life.

Conscious recognition that women were tearing up the deal began with Friedan's exposure of the problem that has no name (1963). She explored the discontent of housewives who appeared to have everything women could want; that is, successful husbands, beautiful children and homes. In Britain, Hannah Gavron found the same responses among working- and middle-class women (1966). Women were no longer content with reduced numbers of pregnancies and live births in exchange for lifelong (or for so long as desired) sexual and domestic services through marriage (or otherwise) to men. But the issues were not formulated in this way.

In the early days the women's liberation movement viewed motherhood, like being a wife, as an oppression, as standing between discovering 'Who am I?' and 'What is a woman?'. It was considered better never to have succumbed to childbearing and rearing, nor to marriage, as being a wife or a mother impeded the development of the consciousness necessary to become autonomous from the male definition of women and his demands. Women who had already succumbed charged other women not to. And in the heady days of the late 1960s and early 1970s childbearing equalled childrearing and so was seen as a drag. The view that women are not 'real women' until they marry and have children was vigorously denied. The 'naturalness' of these female roles was rejected and defined as idology buttressing the exploitation of women.

In terms of action, biological reproduction remained linked to childrearing in the women's liberation movement, although everyone recognized that through fostering, adoption, nurseries and other forms of collective childcare, they could be split. The desirability of relieving women of full-time childcare was enshrined in one of the first four demands made by the women's liberation movement in 1970: twenty-four-hour nurseries on demand. The aim was to give women more choice in how they spent their time and with whom, in order to enable women to gain more control over their lives (New and David 1985).

The major slogan of the women's liberation movement is a demand for control over our bodies. Initially this referred not so much to sexuality or childcare as to biological reproduction, and in particular, abortion. For some women liberation was interpreted as being absolutely certain that heterosexuality would not result in children. Other women were (ana are) still being forced to have children they do not want by being denied effective access to contraception or by being given dangerous contraceptives. Further, before the disaster of thalidomide radically altered public opinion, women also were deprived of legal access to abortion in Britain. Later the problem that some women are being denied the opportunity to have children was recognized and opposition to forced sterilization was added to the demand for abortion within the National Abortion Campaign.

At the same time pregnancy and birth were being increasingly managed through technological means – from an increase in antenatal testing to an increase in mechanical foetal monitoring and deliveries through Caesarians and forceps. The hospital antenatal treatment and the process of birth began to be challenged by other women through demands for 'natural' childbirth classes and deliveries. Growing demands for home confinements with midwives in attendance paralleled the lessening numbers of women who bear children in these conditions, although highly motivated and confident women can sometimes achieve the birth conditions of their choice.

The ways in which medical practice police women began to be explored historically. Ehrenreich and English described the process by which women were driven out of their central role as healers with the growth of modern medicine and its professional hierarchy (1978). The reduction of women to helpmates of male doctors began to be documented, adding fuel to the demand for a woman-centred medicine and practice (Brighton Women and Science Group 1980; and Oakley 1985).

Today the problem among feminists has become how to achieve voluntary childbearing and how to overcome involuntary childlessness or infertility. The recognition grows that women's reproductive processes are being taken over, by being controlled more closely at every stage, if not ultimately to be replaced by artificial machinery to gestate the young. The threat is that women's experience of reproduction may become as discontinuous as that of men.

But the first of the new technologies altering the process of conception, artificial insemination by husband (AIH) or by donor (AID), is not highly technical. In 1960 a British government committee appointed to investigate artificial insemination accepted AIH but strongly opposed the use of AID by unmarried women (lesbians were unmentionable then), and would have recommended making the practice illegal if it had been enforceable (Feversham Committee 1960 and Hanmer 1981). However, because they feared that publicity would encourage the use of AID, they left it to the discretion of the medical profession, labelling the technique an infertility treatment.

But artificial insemination furthered choice for some women. Becoming a lesbian no longer meant the automatic renunciation of pregnancy, birth and having a child with whom to share life. The biological father might or might not be know, and it is the woman who can make the decision. Women joined with others to establish self-insemination groups, obtaining sperm from friends, often gay men (Feminist Self-Insemination Group 1980; Hornstein 1984; and Duelli Klein 1984). Today every major city in Britain has at least one self-insemination group and the oldest children are now in school.

However, we should not assume that women can so easily acquire the knowledge necessary to turn the later increasingly 'high tech' interventions to our advantage, nor even retain our access to AID. The British government committee of today, with more technologies to consider (*in vitro* fertilization, embryo replacement, embryo transfer, embryo freezing and the promise of much more – cloning, sex selection, ectogenesis) looks for new ways of controlling access. The Warnock Report (1984) recommends that the new technologies, including artificial insemination, should be made available only to heterosexual *couples* in stable relationships, married or otherwise. Consent for use by a women should be gained from the husband or cohabitee. They should not be available to the single woman, the one-parent mother, the lesbian. The proposed 'licensing authority' backed up by a series of new criminal offences will ensure 'proper use'.

Women are perceived as having a role to play in raising the young as long as they are dependent on husband or cohabitee for receipt of sperm, for conception, aided by the professional when and how necessary to ensure 'safe' maternal environments and deliveries of 'perfect' babies. At the heart of the Warnock Report is the message that nothing need change between men and women; their power over us is to remain intact. Their overt concern is with embryos and with the family, and not women, the childbearers, who are rarely mentioned.

That men identify with embryos and foetuses, and not mothers, is clear from the debates on abortion rights and, more recently, the Warnock recommendations and parliamentary response to limiting experimentation on human embryos (House of Commons 1984; House of Lords 1984; and Powell Bill 1985). Men also identify with the family, a euphemism for a system of legally defined relations between men and women governing the access of men to women and their labour including all the aspects discussed here. Women are rarely mentioned in the Warnock Report as they are subsumed within men's identification as embryos, foetuses, children and men within the family.

Surrogacy is the second issue to be taken up by parliament as an emergency response to the Warnock Report. *In vitro* fertilization opens up the possibility of surrogacy in which eggs are transferred from one woman to another. The more publicized situation is when a woman bears a child for a couple with the husband's sperm. The outcry against surrogacy in Britain is interesting. No doubt women can be abused by the spread of this practice, but surrogacy, like AID, can put power in women's hands. Could this explain the vehemence of the opposition to *all* surrogacy, not just the money-making agencies?

The implied message of the media as well as the Warnock Report is that technology is best and can do the job of reproduction better than women can on their own. Men, through their technology, can perfect embryos, ensure perfect pregnancies and deliveries. Women, with only their crude bodies, cannot. This message tears at female consciousness and identity. Reproductive technologies remove the last woman-centred process from us. Women who are past childbearing can feel relief at being spared this future. Women of childbearing age whose reproductive consciousness was moulded in an earlier decade may try to carefully tread their way through the worst linguistic abuses; from 'lab parents' to 'father of the century' to describe the largely male medical role in IVF (Corea 1985 and *Guardian* 1983). We *know* in the deepest layers of our selves that they are not the parents or a super father far more important than a mere mother.

But what of the consciousness and identity of women to come? What of women being born today who in twenty years time will sit in front of the white-coated professional, whose array of interventions has grown daily, being assessed for suitability to birth 'naturally'; for suitability to produce 'normal' or 'perfect' offspring? Will women at last be reduced to the receptacle St Thomas Aquinas described – with the lab-coated professionals providing the homunculus, the little man he believed to be intact in the male seed? Will all that *really* matters, the sperm, egg, embryos, be supplied by the 'storage authority', the linguistic invention of the Warnock Committee? Or possibly women will be assessed as unsuitable even for that – a defective maternal environment best replaced by the glass womb (Hubbard 1984). 'It will be safer/better for your baby, Mrs A.' 'You don't want to take any risks, do you, Mrs A.' Will the category of handicap be expanded to include more and more characteristics shared by an ever-increasing proportion of the population – for example, short-sightedness or allergies? (Saxton 1984).

The new reproductive technologies and their control by the state are subtly altering the consciousness of women. The power of the penis is literally and metaphorically strengthened through tighter control over the lives of women. The women already grateful for the gift of life, if not to her individual husband then to the power of professionals dominated by men whose power is consolidated in the state, will bend her knee even further in gratitude. For we are talking about treatments for infertility are we not? How are we to stop this glib lie in order to ensure that this is not the future of our daughters and all the daughters' daughters to come?

I have been discussing women's reproductive consciousness as if all women will be affected in the same way and to the same extent. This is unlikely to be so as colour, culture, country of origin, disability, sexuality, religion and age are factors likely to affect inequality in response to women. We must assume that women will be divided against each other with some receiving preferential treatment, whatever that proves to be. Possibly there will be fine gradations of differential use as divide and conquer remains one of the best tactics in maintaining control in any exploitative system.

A differential response to women is almost certain to occur world wide as well as within national boundaries. Even if the worst abuses are controlled in Britain, for example, scientific experimentation can be taken into the so-called Third World as the new reproductive technologies are international developments. Plans are underway to use women from poorer countries as surrogates (Corea 1985). People in these countries sell their body parts for First World use; for example, one of their kidneys, so why not the eggs and wombs of women? Why not perfect techniques outlawed in the First World in the so-called Third World? We have only to remember the use of Puerto Rican women to develop hormonal contraception to recognize the likelihood of this.

Whatever happens to biological reproduction, working-class and any other category of men will not be affected as much as working-class and any other category of women. The role of biological reproduction for women is far greater, both literally and in terms of the meaning it has for being female or male. Even if the genetic material of their men were not used, the control of women's reproduction furthers the power of working-class and any other category of men over their wives by demonstrating the power of men *per se* to determine which egg, which sperm, which sex, when, and how often she may bear the new generation, if indeed she is allowed to do so at all. In these ways socially powerful men have class interests with socially non-powerful men.

Men as a social group are pressing relentlessly on to the terrain of women's identity and consciousness. Will the day arrive when women painfully try to recreate a sense of ourselves as reproducers of the young – or valid reproducers – as we have witnessed over the past fifteen years in our struggle to create a woman-centred sexual identity and consciousness? The comparison allows us to begin to count the emotional cost that ever lessening security of identity brings.

As McKinnon sums it up, through the structuring of sexuality women and men are divided into genders, while heterosexuality institutionalizes male sexual dominance and female sexual submission (McKinnon 1982). The question then becomes, if women's sexuality is the capacity to arouse desire in the male, is women's sexuality ('true' sexuality) its absence?

> If women are socially defined such that female sexuality cannot be lived or spoken or felt or even somatically sensed apart from its enforced definition, so that it *is* its own lack, then there is no such thing as a woman as such, there are only walking embodiments of men's projected needs. For feminism, asking whether there is, socially, a female sexuality is the same as asking whether women exist. (p. 20.)

McKinnon argues that to be deprived of one's sexuality is to be deprived of selfhood. If biological reproduction becomes ever more securely the gift of men, how will the taking away of a process hardly ever questioned, given its believed timeless 'natural' quality, add to this loss of self?

Biological reproduction, children, and mothering have given rise to a number of theoretical questions that attempt to locate the basis of women's oppression; to answer, 'Who is the oppressor and why?' Is male envy of women's role in reproducing the new generation the cause of women's oppression by men? Widely discussed in the early days of the women's liberation movement and criticized for being an explanation based on biology, it was finally dismissed by Shulamith Firestone who found it unbelievable that anyone would *want* to bear babies (1971).

Is it children themselves that oppress women? The most popularized version of this view identifies the social isolation of women with children, particularly when under 5 years of age, as the problem (Barrett and McIntosh 1982). The discussion turns on how to make childrearing less isolating an experience. Then Adrienne Rich lifted theory into the world of social relations by conceptualizing motherhood as a social institution as well as a personal experience (Rich 1976). The institution has many elements; legal, economic, cultural and psychological, through which women's oppression is organized and her resistance takes form. But locating the issue solely in the social isolation of mothers neatly sidesteps a closer look at the institution as a whole and at the question of who determines these conditions and why.

The experience of motherhood as resistance to male power and the expression of human feeling so beautifully expressed by Rich is transformed by the question 'Is it because women mother that they are oppressed by men?' Dinnerstein argues that the experience of helplessness when an infant gives rise to the male need to control women later in life (1977), while Chodorow sees the oppression of women arising from the impact of mothering on the complex relation between the social and the psychological in gender role formation (1978). However unintentionally, it is women, ourselves, who create the conditions for our oppression.

The most frequently voiced solution to these questions is to give men a greater role in childrearing. In this way men are to be humanized and women released from unremitting toil so that they too can develop their full range of human qualities. Shulamith Firestone's desire to free women from biological reproduction is achieved in the utopia of Marge Piercy. Both men and women nurse and care for the children born of the glass womb (1976). The new deal between men and women becomes – 'we will help you if you give up your special role' – and it works in fiction.

Meanwhile, back in today's reality, women continue to carry the main burden of childcare (Boulton 1984). Studies of housework show that in socialist and capitalist societies alike, women are the unpaid and overworked workers of the world. Further, women who share childcare with men are more vulnerable to losing contested custody cases in the increasing number of marriages that end in divorce. It is not necessary to be a lesbian to lose one's children; reading *Spare Rib* and sharing childcare can be sufficient (Rights of Women 1984; and Smart 1984).

Shared childcare as a solution to women's oppression is based on a belief that there are no serious contradictions between men and women (Ehrensaft 1980; and Riley 1983). Re-education is the means of dealing with contradictions *among* the people – unlike those *between* the people which require real winners and real losers, i.e. the class revolution (Mao 1966). Those who see shared childcare as the solution argue that the reasons men should want to take on more work in an already full day is because they will be better people for it, more developed emotionally, more capable of relationships of warmth and love. Betty Friedan, for example, believes this has already happened (1983). For those who know it has not, proposed solutions are shorter working days, job sharing and part-time work (Phillips 1983). But no matter how intense the re-education, men are not rushing to relieve women of their labour in sufficient number to alter the depressing statistics on women's paid and unpaid working hours relative to those of men.

Mary O'Brien also argues for shared childcare, but from theory based on biology utilizing a Hegelian/Marxist tradition (O'Brien 1981 and 1982). The question arising from her work can be phrased, 'Is it because men experience their role in reproduction as alienating that women are oppressed?' While acknowledging her debt to Marx, she argues that Marxism cannot explain the oppression of women which transcends class. O'Brien uses the concept of dialectics which insists that the structure of consciousness proceeds from the negation of alienation. She attempts to show that the negation of alienation arising out of the male reproductive experience is the motor force structuring the history of male–female relations. She argues that for men, reproductive consciousness is a discontinuous process, while for women there is a continuity from conception, to gestation, to birth. She contends that this discontinuity, due to the discovery by men of their role in biological reproduction at some unknown historical time, fuels men's desire to achieve continuity.

Mary O'Brien is arguing from biology, and this is essential to her theory. But it does not matter if men's view of their role in reproduction as discontinuous is 'natural' or socially constructed, as long as it is interpreted in this way by men. Either way the logical conclusion is for the male to find ways of ensuring that he *is* the father. *In vitro* fertilization gives absolute certainty in a way that conception via intercourse cannot. Further, *in vitro* fertilization creates uncertainty about who the mother is. The present biological uncertainty of fatherhood in reproduction via intercourse is exchanged, or at least equated. Her egg, removed from her, must be returned; creating room for doubt, error and abuse. 'Lab parents' fill the vacuum. The mother is devalued; her biological certainty that this is *her* child dissolves on several layers of consciousness.

Mediation of men's alienation can be achieved by their progressive intervention into women's biological productive processes, but O'Brien chooses to argue mediation through equality in childcare. In Marxism human labour is needed to overcome alienation. But why not overcome male alienation through scientific enterprises to replicate women's biological processes, particularly as men and women's certainty in conception can be exchanged? Why need alienation be overcome through childcare?

Mary O'Brien argues that motherhood has been a duty without rights and is about to become a major political issue. As a result, parenthood may become an 'authentic human and social project'; one that is 'freely chosen and rationally controlled' (1982: p. 110). The new model must recognize that production and reproduction are necessary substructures of human survival. For O'Brien this means integration of women on equal terms in the productive realm and integration of men into relations of reproduction and active care of the next generation. While recognizing that 'male potency is an amalgam of the power to appropriate, supported by the socially bestowed right to do so, and dependent on suspicious co-operation between men', she does not suggest any necessary reason why men should give up their power over women in exchange for equality with us (1982: p. 109).

There is nothing intrinsically 'natural' about the experience of childcare. Its desirability and organization could be profoundly altered within male-dominated social structures once biological reproduction is completely understood. Childcare, like sexuality, could be taken from women either completely or through the even more exact shaping of social roles and experience. Women could become even more like servants than today. The analogy could be the black nursemaid of apartheid systems from the USA to South Africa, often loved but always denied. How is this scenario to be avoided?

Mary O'Brien believes that men 'can only be disarmed when women experience a change in reproductive consciousness comparable in scope to the discovery of paternity' (1982: p. 108). She sees this happening if women are truly able to control their reproductive processes so that reproduction for women is transformed from involuntary labour to voluntary labour. Voluntary reproductive labour is not defined, however. Is this being able to choose with the consent of one's husband (and possibly the state, as in China) that this year I will have a child? Or is true voluntary reproductive labour being able to decide that this year I will have a child with or without a known father (and without the intervention of the state)? This latter is what happens with self-insemination by lesbians and heterosexual women who do not want a known father around, and the rejection of this by the state is evident in the Warnock Report, for example.

For other women there can hardly be said to be a choice given the strength of heterosexuality as a social institution. By and large a woman does not question whether or not there should be a known father 'legitimating' the child through his status as husband. Her control over reproduction is largely a farce. At most it will lie in deciding, with her husband's agreement, that this year is a suitable one for having a child. We can argue that when there is no contraception this is better than being at the mercy of her own and her husband's fertility. But what if he decides he does not want any children, or has decided she should have another now, or some particular number? While individuals may be better, or worse off in that personalities can make an impact – overall we are discussing 'choice' in a context of individual and social male domination as O'Brien clearly recognizes.

Women have a continuous biological experience from providing a sex cell to conception to pregnancy to birth. To interrupt this by taking away one or more processes would disrupt consciousness as the *potential* is there. The parallel is sexuality. Women have the physical capacity for sexual pleasure. To deny it individually and culturally is experienced as a lack and as an undermining of the self. If men experience their biological role in reproduction as discontinuous this is more likely to be a cultural phenomenon connected with the acquisition of personal and social power, as none of their biology is being denied. The alternative explanation, of course, is that their biology *is* inferior, and they know it, hence their active striving to gain control of women's wombs (Al-Hibri 1983).

With rape the first question posed is whether it is violence or sexuality that motivates the aggressor male. Rephrased from the point of view of women, rape is always about sexuality (McKinnon 1983). Perceiving rape entails reclaiming sexuality as something that does not exist in and for men, as men cannot take what is already theirs. If female sexuality already belongs to men, in that it does not exist except in reference to them, then men cannot be guilty of rape as it must be something the woman has done – her dress, behaviour, past. This is the response of the criminal justice system to allegations of rape, as we know.

Is this response also happening in relation to female biological reproduction? Men already feel they have a right to women's eggs and, as they are more likely to experiment upon women than men, it can be inferred that women are seen as more suitable for medical experimentation. The issue of informed consent is slid over easily. It is not even recognized as a problem in the Warnock Report, for example. How much more securely men will feel that biological reproduction belongs solely to them once ectogenesis is perfected. The flip side of this control is a belief that they can do as they please with women's actual bodies as they already own them – 'You can't take that which already belongs to you.'

The separation of heterosexuality from reproduction begins with contraception and abortion and ends with ectogenesis. Despite the power of individual men, morality and marriage are no longer effective controllers of the expression of sexuality and thereby biological reproduction. The dominant mode of control is changing hands from the individual male through marriage to men as a social category, through science and technology, and the pace is accelerating. The locus of control and struggle is shifting from sexuality to reproduction and childcare, i.e. motherhood.

Women are being policed by the shaping of the role 'fit mother'. Motherhood is being more tightly structured; to be a 'fit mother' is a more carefully defined concept. It is monitored from antenatal care onwards and involves medical personnel, health visitors, teachers, social workers, social security, housing and legal workers. The state directly shapes and supervises the 'fit mother' as concept and individual through the personal social services, social security, housing, the health service, education, law and the legal system. Reproductive technology offers the possibility to extend the shaping of the 'fit mother' to include the 'fit reproducer'. The state is directly involved through its support for, and control of, science and technology. There is no corresponding 'fit father' role.

The taking of independent actions within biological reproduction and childcare away from women is not really recognized as the major issue. Seeing the solution as shared childcare, or believing reproductive technology to be about overcoming infertility, locates the problem in women as biological and social mothers. To do so ignores the extension of 'rights' and power over women as *mothers* by men, both individually and as a social category.

Is there a male conspiracy? There is a massive cover-up of the effects of contraception and its relation to cancer and infertility. Perhaps there is a professional conspiracy, however well intended. But then the pharmaceutical companies are also involved in the failure to inform the public. The promoters of reproductive technology do not need a conspiracy in the sense that 'we will make them do something they do not want to do' as sufficient women volunteer for these so-called treatments in the hope of a child. Women, like men, can be blinded by science and technology. This should come as no surprise as the shaping of women to be responsive to the desires of the medical and scientific worlds is rarely challenged. The situation in which we women find ourselves is far more serious than conscious conspiracy which always implies that most people will disagree once the evil plotters are discovered.

We live in a social climate and in an intellectual tradition in which violence and sexuality are conflated; man the aggressor pursues woman the masochistic victim. Women's bodies become the nature to be controlled (Easlea 1983). In cultures that prize individual competition and money-making there are personal advancements and financial spin-offs. For example, there are patents on certain *in vitro* fertilization procedures developed at the University of Melbourne in Australia, and sex predetermination techniques are marketed in the USA.

To define these issues as being about women's 'choice' and 'rights' is totally inadequate, as these concepts are based on liberal philosophy in which there are no serious differences in interests or power between social groups that make up society. While this response is also inadequate for earlier interventions in biological reproduction (Pollock 1984), the new technologies expose the politics of male supremacy far more clearly. We need to rediscuss motherhood, biological reproduction, childcare and the relation of these to sexuality and the personhood of women, bearing in mind that we live in a gendered society in which women are subordinate. The discussion thus far has been too superficial. The totality of the control of women's bodies which is now becoming feasible alters the terms in which the new reproductive technologies must be considered.

The defence of women's potential and real power in the reproductive process may seem to be a reactionary argument to some, particularly given the struggle in the early days of the women's liberation movement to remove 'natural' elements from our consciousness of 'What is a woman?'. But we are not in a position to determine the direction of science or technology, nor do we control their empowerment through incorporation in the state. Therefore we must resist the use of science and technology to further shape women; our consciousness, our behaviour, and assumptions about who we are.

As we know, socially powerful groups can more easily manipulate both belief systems and material conditions than can less powerful groups, together or separately, depending upon the nature of the threat to their power. Subordinate groups have to overthrow dominant ideas as well as social practices in order to be heard and seen. Recent feminist analysis tends to see biological reproduction and childcare as a consequence of heterosexuality both as a sexual act and as a system of social relations (Rich 1980; McKinnon 1983). But heterosexuality need not result in children, and women can have children without heterosexual sex. By organizing separately around sexuality, biological reproduction and childcare, women have demonstrated these aspects of women's lives to be experientially distinct.

We need to consider why biological reproduction is being modified now and how this relates to other aspects of women's lives. Sexuality, reproduction and childcare are related in that the superordinate always has the advantage and can call the shots, so to speak. An attack in one area can be answered by an offensive in another. Sexuality, reproduction and childcare all belong in the 'private' sphere, the sphere of women's subordination. However hypothesized, as labour relations or power relations, women create products in the private sphere in which men can take more than they give. As women make a sustained attack on male sexuality as a form of colonization of women, and a few women are even refusing to serve, the present wave of the women's movement is helping to tear up the deal, i.e. lifelong service to men in exchange for limited pregnancies and births. I argue that the counter-attack is a tightening control over female reproductive processes and motherhood.

But the Establishment is treading on dangerous grounds, too. If the deal has been torn up, where will it all end? It is almost as if the British government's Warnock Committee knew this, hence their concern with serving the 'family', by creating 'perfect' babies for 'perfect' couples. The denial of what is going on is tearing the roots of society itself – unbalancing even further the unequal relationship between men and women. If they take reproduction from us, what do they want next? An even more enslaved caste? Our lives? As technology is used to undermine us, transforming our consciousness of ourselves as even more inferior to men than it is today, in consciousness lies our only defence.

P.S. At last I have discovered what the term mother-fucker means and who the mother-fuckers are. For years I have wondered what this ultimate of oaths, the most serious swear word in the American lexicon was about.

References

Al-Hibra, Azizah, 'Reproduction, Mothering and the Origins of Patriarchy', in Trebilcot, Joyce (ed.), *Mothering: Essays in Feminist Theory* (NJ: Rowman & Allanheld 1983).

Arditti, Rita, Duelli Klein, Renate, and Minden, Shelley (eds), *Test-Tube Women. What future for motherhood?* (London and Boston: Pandora Press 1984).

Barrett, Michele, and McIntosh, Mary, *The Anti-Social Family* (London: Verso 1982).

Bartky, Sandra Lee, 'Towards a phenomenology of feminist consciousness', in Vetterling-Braggin, Mary, Elliston, Frederick, and English, Jane (eds), *Feminism and Philosophy* (NJ: Littlefield, Adams 1977).

The Brighton Women and Science Group, *Alice Through the Microscope: the power of science over women's lives* (London: Virago 1980).

Brunt, Rosalind, and Rowan, Caroline (eds), *Feminism, Culture and Politics* (London: Lawrence & Wishart 1982).

Boulton, Mary, *On Being A Mother* (London: Methuen 1984).

Chodorow, Nancy, *The Reproduction of Mothering: Psychoanalysis and the sociology of gender* (Berkeley: University of California Press 1978).

Coveney, Lal, Jackson, Margaret, Jeffreys, Sheila, Kay, Leslie, and Mahony, Pat, *The Sexuality Papers: Male sexuality and the social control of women* (London: Hutchinson 1984).

Corea, Genoveffa, *The Mother Machine: Reproductive technologies from artificial insemination to artificial wombs* (NY: Harper and Row 1985).
David, Miriam, and New, Caroline, *For the Children's Sake: Making Childcare more than Women's Business* (Harmondsworth: Penguin 1985).
Davies, Margaret Llewelyn (ed.) (1915), *Maternity: Letters from Working Women* (London: Virago 1978).
Dinnerstein, Dorothy, *The Mermaid and the Minotaur: Sexual arrangements and human malaise* (NY: Harper and Row 1976; London: Souvenir Press (Condor Books) 1978; retitled: *The Rocking of the Cradle, and the Ruling of the World*).
Duelli Klein, Renate, 'Doing It Ourselves: Self-Insemination', in Arditti *et al.*, *Test-Tube Women* (1984), pp. 382–90.
Ehrensaft, Diane, 'When Women and Men Mother', *Politics & Power* (3) (1980) (London: Routledge & Kegan Paul 1981), pp. 21–47.
Easlea, Brian, *Fathering the Unthinkable: Masculinity, scientists and the nuclear arms race* (London: Pluto 1983).
Ehrenreich, Barbara, and English, Deidre, *For Her Own Good: 150 years of the experts' advice to women* (Garden City, NY: Anchor Press/Doubleday 1978).
Faderman, Lilian, *Surpassing the Love of Man: Romantic Friendship & Loves between women from the Renaissance to the Present* (London: Junction Books 1981).
Feversham Committee, *The Report of the Departmental Committee on Human Artificial Insemination*, Cmnd 1105 (London: HMSO 1960).
Feminist Self-Insemination Group (1980), *Self-Insemination*, PO Box No. 3, 190 Upper Street, London, N1, UK.
Friedan, Nancy, *The Feminist Mystique* (1963; repr. Harmondsworth: Penguin 1965).
Friedan, Nancy, *The Second Stage* (London: Michael Joseph 1982).
Firestone, Shulamith, *The Dialetic of Sex: The case for feminist revolution* (London: Jonathan Cape 1971).
Gavron, Hannah, *The Captive Wife: Conflicts of housebound mothers* (1966; repr. London: Routledge & Kegan Paul 1983).
Guardian, 'Father of the Century' (25 June 1983).
Hanmer, Jalna, 'Sex predetermination, artificial insemination and the maintenance of male dominated culture', in Roberts, Helen (ed.), *Women, Health & Reproduction* (London: Routledge & Kegan Paul 1981).
Hornstein, Francie, 'Children by donor insemination: a new choice for lesbians', in Arditti, *et al.*, *Test-Tube Women* (1984), pp. 373–81.

House of Commons Parliamentary Debates (Friday, 23 November 1984), *Hansard,* Vol. 68, No. 14 (London: HMSO), pp. 528–90.

House of Commons, *Unborn Children (Protection) Bill* (The Powell Bill), 1985.

House of Lords Parliamentary Debates (Wednesday, 31 October 1984), Vol. 456, No. 180 (London: HMSO), pp. 524–31.

Hubbard, Ruth, 'Personal Courage is not Enough: Some hazards of child bearing in the 1980's', in Arditti, *et al., Test-Tube Women* (1984), pp. 331–55.

Jeffreys, Sheila, '"Free from all uninvited touch of man": women's campaigns around sexuality 1880–1914', *Women's Studies International Forum,* 5 (6) (1982), and Coveney, *et al., The Sexuality Papers* (1984).

Johnston, Jill, *Lesbian Nation: The feminist solution* (NY: Simon & Schuster 1973).

McLaren, Angus, *Reproductive Rituals* (London: Methuen 1984).

McKinnon, Catherine, 'Feminism, Marxism, Method and the State: an agenda for theory', *SIGNS,* 7 (3) (1982), pp. 515–44.

McKinnon, Catherine, 'Feminism, Marxism, Method and the State: towards feminist jurisprudence', *SIGNS,* 8 (4) (1983), pp. 635–58.

Mao Tse-Tung, *Four Essays on Philosophy* (Peking: Foreign Languages Press 1966).

Masters, William, and Johnson, Virginia, *Human Sexual Response* (Boston: Little Brown 1966).

O'Brien, Mary, *The Politics of Reproduction* (London: Routledge & Kegan Paul 1981).

O'Brien, Mary, 'Feminist theory and Dialectical Logic', in Keohane, Namnerl, Rosaldo, Michelle, and Gelpi, Barbara (eds), *Feminist Theory: A critique of ideology* (Brighton: Harvester Press 1982), pp. 99–112.

Oakley, Ann, *Captured Womb: History of the medical care of pregnant women* (Oxford: Blackwell 1985).

Phillips, Anne, *Hidden Hands: Women and economic policies* (London: Pluto 1983).

Piercy, Marge, *Women on the Edge of Time* (NY: Knopf 1976; London: Women's Press 1978).

Pollock, Scarlet, 'Refusing to Take Women Seriously: "Side effects" and the politics of contraception', in Arditti, *et al., Test-Tube Women* (1984), pp. 138–52.

Rich, Adrienne, *Of Woman Born – Motherhood as experience and institution* (London: Virago 1977).

Rich, Adrienne, 'Compulsory Heterosexuality and Lesbian Existence', *SIGNS*, 5 (4) (1980), pp. 631–60.

Rights of Women, *Lesbian Mothers on Trial: A report on lesbian mothers and child custody* (London: ROW 1984).

Smart, Carole, *The Ties that Bind: Law, marriage and the reproduction of patriarchal relations* (London: Routledge & Kegan Paul 1984).

Riley, Denise, 'The Serious Burdens of Love', in Segal, Lynne (ed.), *What is to be Done About the Family?* (Harmondsworth: Penguin 1983).

Saxton, Marsha, 'Born and Unborn: the implications of reproductive technologies for people with disabilities', in Arditti, *et al.*, *Test-Tube Women* (1984), pp. 298–312.

Warnock Committee, *Report of the Committee of Inquiry into Human Fertilisation and Embryology*, Cmnd 9314 (London: HMSO 1984).

Warnock, Mary, *A Question of Life: The Warnock Report on human fertilisation and embryology* (Oxford: Basil Blackwell 1985).

Note

I would like to thank Gena Corea for giving me back the idea for this article, Renate Duelli Klein for constant encouragement ('You will do it, won't you, Jalna'), Miriam David, Deena Attar and two wonderful women's meetings in London and York for helpful comments and insights, and the FINNRET network for extending the possibility of challenge.